Basics of Chimeric Antigen Receptor (CAR) Immunotherapy

Basics of Chimeric Antigen Receptor (CAR) Immunotherapy

MUMTAZ YASEEN BALKHI, PH.D.,

Scientific Director
Immunotherapy, Immune Therapy Bio (IT Bio, LLC), Cambridge
Massachusetts, United States
Assistant Professor
Medicine, Tufts University School of Medicine, BOSTON
Massachusetts, United States
Assistant Professor (cooperating)
Molecular and Biomedical Sciences
University of Maine, Orono, Maine, United States

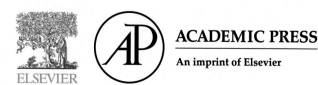

ELSEVIER

ACADEMIC PRESS
An imprint of Elsevier

Basics of Chimeric Antigen Receptor (CAR) Immunotherapy

ISBN: 978-0-12-819573-4

Copyright © 2020 Elsevier Inc. All rights reserved.

Notices

Publisher: Andre G. Wolff
Acquisition Editor: Linda Versteeg-buschman
Editorial Project Manager: Rebeka Henry
Production Project Manager: Poulouse Joseph
Cover Designer: Alan Studholme

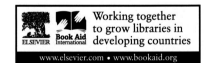

Working together to grow libraries in developing countries

www.elsevier.com • www.bookaid.org

Preface

T-cell adoptive immunotherapy has power to cure metastatic malignant cancers. The recent clinical data obtained with the checkpoint receptor blockade inhibitory drugs and chimeric antigen receptor (CAR)-T cell therapy have been promising. The success of these therapies have generated renewed hope that we may be finally at the verge of not only treating but curing the cancer. Cancer is a disease that is synonymous with death attached to a time lens, that is, death is destined subject to overall survival rates. This makes cancer a dreadful disease. Over the years, huge progress has been made in controlling and in some rare cases actually "curing" the stage IV-metastasized cancers through clinical application of checkpoint receptor inhibitory drugs and CAR therapy. These interventions have generated unprecedented interest in immunotherapy field. Very deservedly, Science magazine chose to celebrate year 2013 as a breakthrough year in cancer immunotherapy [1,2]. Another important milestone that CAR therapy achieved was gaining the Food and Drug Administration (FDA) approval of first ever CAR therapy product Kymriah (tisagenlecleucel) [3] and Yescarta (axicabtagene ciloleucel) [4] for the treatment of refractory B cell acute lymphoblastic leukemia (B cell-ALL) and diffuse large B cell lymphoma (DLBCL). With FDA approval of the first CARs, promise of these therapies have been firmly established, and the excitement generated thereof has reached far and wide. I felt there was tremendous need for the book on CAR-Immunotherapy that succinctly elaborate fundamental concepts and molecular biology approaches being applied in designing CAR immunotherapy, and concurrently provide readers with new knowledge and highlight latest advancements being made in the field. The target audience for this book are students and biomedical researchers who will greatly benefit from the in-depth discussion and wide range of CAR-immunotherapy topics covered in the book. Several universities have already begun to introduce courses that incorporate immunotherapy as part of introductory immunology courses. Therefore, keeping in mind the general interest of students, postdoctoral fellows, clinical scientists, and biomedical researchers, I begin this book by providing a historical narrative that led to the present breakthrough in CAR therapy. This is followed by in-depth discussion on the immune escape mechanisms that led to the concept of targeting immune escape through CARs. We provide thorough understanding on how chimeric genes especially single-chain variable fragments are selected, cloned, expressed, and tested in vitro and in vivo in preclinical models. A comprehensive protocol is provided for the preclinical production of CARs. CARs produced preclinically are utilized for the in vitro testing in laboratories and for in vivo testing in animal models. A full chapter is devoted to discussing various clinical protocols utilized to conduct actual clinical trials with CARs. CARs have shown remarkable success in eradicating B-cell malignancies but the success rate against solid cancers have been low. In the final chapter of the book, we discuss various challenges facing the CAR therapy and explore the underlying mechanisms leading to CAR-T cell dysfunction in solid cancers. Accordingly, we thoroughly discuss on-target/off-tumor toxicity, cytokine storm syndrome, neurological pathologies, and contingency plans that are put in place to mitigate these toxicities. We discuss some of the novel concepts that have been tested to minimize CAR-related toxicities without compromising their efficacy. One such concept that we discuss in detail is related to dual CAR expression in a T cell in which one CAR senses tumor antigen and sends signal to the second CAR to help redirect CARs to the tumor-rich environment to perform tumor lysis, and this mechanism has potential to greatly minimize the off-tumor toxicities. Finally, we elaborate on the challenges and promises of "Universal-off-the-shelf CARs" that if successful could benefit large number of cancer patients including those who otherwise cannot afford the costly autologous CAR-therapy treatment. I envision CAR therapy to be retaining almost the same status as bone marrow transplantation with perhaps every hospital in the country and around the world someday having separate CAR-therapy units dedicated to treat cancers.

REFERENCES

[1] Couzin-Frankel J. Breakthrough of the year 2013. Cancer immunotherapy Science 2013;342:1432–3.

[2] Eshhar Z. From the mouse cage to human therapy: a personal perspective of the emergence of T-bodies/chimeric antigen receptor T cells. Hum Gene Ther 2014;25:773–8.

[3] FDA. The FDA approved Kymriah (tisagenlecleucel). 2017.

[4] FDA. FDA Approved Yescarta (axicabtagene ciloleucel). 2018.

Contents

CHAPTER 1

An Introduction to CAR Immunotherapy

IMMUNOTHERAPY: HISTORICAL PERSPECTIVE

The concept that human immune system has a power to protect from diseases especially infections has been in existence for the past 2000 years [1]. The therapeutic potential of immune system was first demonstrated by Edward Jenner who in 1798 applied "rudimentary vaccination-inoculation technique" to treat small pox. Edward Jenner was unknowingly invigorating immune system to eradicate small pox disease, which fits into our definition of immunotherapy. Similarly, Dr. William B. Coley in the late 18th century recognized the power of immune system for curing cancer [2]. Dr. Coley was working with a patient who had recurrent sarcoma growth and had developed an unhealed ulcerated wound after the surgical resection of sarcoma tumor. The patient developed a spontaneous regression of tumor and wound healing after she had contracted *Streptococcus pyogenes* infection [3]. This led Dr. Coley to pioneer an idea of injecting first live bacteria and later a mixture of two killed bacteria into a patient suffering from malignant tumor growth to bring a nonspecific immune activation against tumors [4]. The approach came to be known as Coley's mixed bacterial toxins [5]. As expected, the results of his treatment were mixed of successes and failures. However, it can be safely argued that Dr. William B. Coley deserves to be called the father of modern cancer immunotherapy.

The field of immunotherapy had remained stagnant for many decades. However, due to the pioneering efforts of several scientists, notable among them Dr. Steven A. Rosenberg of National Cancer Institute, USA; Dr. Zelig Eshhar of Weizmann Institute of Sciences, Israel; Dr. James Allison, University of Texas MD Anderson Cancer Center, Houston, USA; Dr. Tasuku Honjo, Kyoto University, Kyoto, Japan, immunotherapy field saw flurry of research activities. These visionary scientists pioneered the renewed interest in immunotherapy field and also contributed toward the remarkable therapeutic success seen with immunotherapy drugs in the last 10 years. It was in late 1980 when Dr. Zelig Eshhar and his team [6,7] came up with a fascinating idea of redirecting T cells to target antigens of choice. The redirection of T cells to target antigens was achieved through cloning a chimeric gene that replaces T-cell receptor (TcRα or TcRβ) variable region with an antibody V_L and V_H region while maintaining the TcR extracellular constant C-region, transmembrane domain, and intracellular signaling domain of T-cell receptor complex. This chimeric receptor that later became popular with the term chimeric antigen receptor or simply CAR provided major histocompatibility (MHC) restriction independent and antibody redirected specificity to such modified T cells. Moreover, these CAR-T cells were also capable of cytokine production when tested in mice [6]. It was quickly recognized that this novel approach had potential to rejuvenate otherwise inert antitumor T-cell responses. However, it took 20 long years before the true potential of the idea of modifying T cells to target tumors was tested successfully in humans. During this time, the prototypical design of chimeric genes and vectors first conceived by Dr. Eshhar and his team underwent several modifications [8].

Almost at the same time when CARs were being designed to engineer T cells to target cancers, Dr. Rosenberg and his team had pioneered a revolutionary concept of treating melanoma patients with adoptive transfer of nonmodified melanoma tumor infiltrating autologous T cells (TILs) and IL2 cytokine [9–12]. Very recently, the usefulness of TILs treatment has been demonstrated in studies that show that TILs can successfully regress melanoma tumors in 70% of patients potentially due to targeting of tumors expressing neoantigens or mutated genes [13,14]. In addition to developing TILs and IL2 treatment for metastatic melanoma, Dr. Rosenberg and his team have been testing to express HLA epitope of tumor antigen—specific TCRs using genetic engineering techniques. Recently, Dr. Rosenberg and his team have envisioned to use nonviral transposon/transposase system to generate tumor antigen—specific TCRs to treat treatment refractive solid tumors and virally induced tumors such as human papilloma virus (HPV) [15,16]. With the advent of high throughput whole exome and RNA-sequencing techniques, it has now become possible to identify neoantigens expressed by solid tumors and

Basics of Chimeric Antigen Receptor (CAR) Immunotherapy. https://doi.org/10.1016/B978-0-12-819573-4.00001-6

also to identify their cognate neoantigen tumor–specific TCRs [16,17]. The key advantage of expressing TCRs is that it allows targeting those solid tumors specifically that accumulate high mutation rates and express neoantigens and, thus, shrink the tumor escape mechanisms [17]. Taken together, the innovative approaches pioneered by the Drs. Zelig Eshhar and Steven Rosenberg have helped to revolutionize the cancer immunotherapy field. Several other eminent scientists among which Nobel laureate Drs. R. Zinkernagel, James Allison, Tasuku Honjo; Drs. Rafi Ahmad, Carl June, Richard P Junghans, Gordon Freeman, and others not named here have been making significant contributions to the immunotherapy field. Their research have proven vital in our understanding of T-cell dysfunction in chronic viral infections and cancer that eventually paved the way for testing, successfully, the checkpoint receptor blockade inhibitory drugs against metastatic cancers. Whether the ongoing research on Immunotherapy can yield immunotherapy-based cure for significant number of cancer patients as well as for other diseases such as chronic viral, bacterial, fungal, parasitic infections, and chronic inflammatory diseases will be revealed in future.

CONCEPTS THAT LED TO THE DEVELOPMENT OF CAR-BASED IMMUNOTHERAPY AGAINST CANCERS

Human immune system is exceptionally efficient to control both infectious and noninfectious diseases. However, cancer is one noninfectious disease that human immune system usually fails to eradicate. There are reports that most tumors express antigens that can be recognized by the T-cell receptors [18]. Yet, antigen specific T cells does not eradicate cancers. The advanced stage cancers such as colorectal, ovarian, and breast cancer in humans, and autochthonous tumors in mice are

T-cell infiltrated [19–22]. Similarly, clinically nonmanifested and noninvasive premalignant latent-stage lesions can induce adaptive immune responses [23]. Yet, despite the T-cell infiltration and effector responses, T cells do not effectively cause the destruction of tumors or prevent latent tumors from progressing aggressively, for example, colorectal tumors that arise from premalignant benign small adenomas transform into metastatic carcinoma that despite colon and small intestine harboring huge number of T cells that according to some estimates number as high as $\sim 3 \times 10^{10}$ [22–26]. The reason immune system fails to eradicate cancers is due to elaborate "immune escape mechanisms" developed by cancers (Fig. 1.1) that help cancers to evade immune recognition, and effector T-cell responses in vivo.

Immune Escape Through Disruption of Antigen Presentation and Costimulation

One of the important immune escape mechanisms may be the deficiency in tumor antigen processing and presentation machinery in tumor cells, those can be collectively referred to as "loss of antigenicity". Antigen processing and presentation is critical in evoking cytolytic T-cell responses against virally infected cells and in malignancy [27]. The MHC Class I-peptide antigen/TCR signaling along with B7/CD28 costimulatory signals are critical for the synthesis of effector cytokines and effector molecules involved in the T-cell-mediated cytolytic activities [28,29]. The description of this process is following: All nucleated cells express MHC-1 molecule including malignant cells [30]. Endogenous antigens are catalytically degraded by the proteasomes especially 26S proteasome in the cytosol. Following their degradation, peptides are transported into endoplasmic reticulum (ER) by the ABC transporter superfamily and the transporter associated with antigen processing TAP-1 and TAP-2 dimer [31]. In the ER

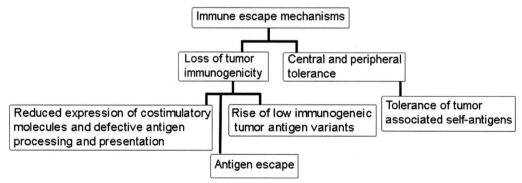

FIG. 1.1 Flow diagram describing various immune escape mechanisms. Loss of tumor immunogenicity and tolerance mechanism are the main barriers to cancer immunotherapy.

antigen peptides bind to the MHC Class 1 molecule peptide-loading complex (PLC). This PLC consists of MHC-1 heavy chain and β2-microglobulin, the adaptor chaperone tapasin, the oxidoreductase ERp57, and lectin-like chaperone calreticulin (Fig. 1.2A) [32]. The tapasin is TAP-associated protein that binds simultaneously to the TAP and MHC-1, thus, plays a role in the assembly and stability of MHC-1 peptide-loading complex in the ER, and assist further in peptide translocation through ER and loading on the MHC-1 peptide-binding cleft [33,34]. The tapasin is also covalently linked with oxidoreductase ERp57 in ER. The Erp57 plays role in antigen processing and is required to maintain integrity of PLC. The chaperone calreticulin reportedly interact with Erp57 and plays a role in MHC-1 peptide loading and presentation on cell surface [32]. Finally, MHC1-peptide complex is released from the ER and transported to Golgi complex before its surface expression and presentation to the T-cell receptors. The MHC1-peptide presentation to the TCR complex in T cells generates membrane proximal events including Lck-mediated phosphorylation of CD3 complex. The phosphorylated tyrosine residues within CD3 dimer complexes, the γε, δε, and ζζ, act as docking sites for other Src homology 2 (SH2) tyrosine kinases, Fyn,

and zeta chain-associated protein (ZAP70). ZAP70 predominantly docks to ITAMs of ζζ dimers (Fig. 1.2A). The binding of ZAP70 to the ITAMs eventually helps its release. The tyrosine residues within ZAP70 are phosphorylated by the Lck or undergo autophosphorylation mediated by ZAP70 itself. Once phosphorylated, ZAP70 drives downstream kinase cascade by directly phosphorylating transmembrane protein linker for activation of T cells (LAT) and SH2 domain-containing leukocyte protein of 76 kDa (SLP76) [35,36]. Both LAT and SLP76 recruit adaptor protein complex Vav, son of sevenless (SOS), growth factor receptor-bound protein 2 (Grb2) that help dispersing TCR signaling from membrane proximal receptor tyrosine kinases. The initial tyrosine phosphorylation events initiates a kinase cascade that activates the transcription factors such as AP1, cJun/ATF2, NFAT, and NF-κB, which are crucial for the synthesis of effector cytokines and effector molecules required for the T-cell cytolytic activities. In addition to the peptide-MHC1/TCR interaction and kinase cascade activation, a second signaling cascade is generated with the B7 and CD28 interactions. The B7/CD28 interaction apart from the serine and threonine resides leads to the phosphorylation of tyrosine residues within CD28 intracellular conserved YMNM motif by the Src

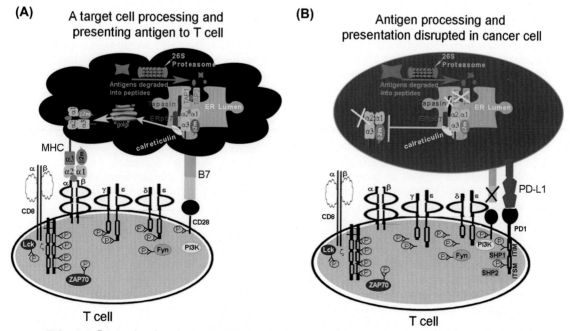

FIG. 1.2 Dysregulated antigen processing and presentation in cancer cells helps to evade immune recognition. **(A)** Important steps involved in antigen processing and presentation to T cells. **(B)** Steps in antigen processing and presentation that gets disrupted in cancer cells because of which T cells can fail to recognize tumor antigens.

family proteins, Fyn and Lck. The phospho-YMNM motif serves as a docking site for the serine-threonine kinase, phosphoinositide 3-kinase (PI3K). The PI3K subsequently phosphorylates AKT to initiate costimulatory signaling cascade that activates transcription factors crucial for cytokine production and T-cell expansion [37,38]. The PI3K-mediated signaling represents predominant signaling cascade initiated with CD28 costimulation [38]. Taken together, the peptide-MHC1/TCR and B7/CD28 interactions are crucial for evoking antitumor T-cell adaptive responses against cancers.

Tumors have evolved various mechanisms to target these two crucial axes for eliciting antitumor responses. Evidences suggest that there is a reduction in the expression of MHC class-I molecules on human tumors [39], for example, melanoma tumors have been reported to lack the MHC-1 beta 2-microglobulin (β2-m) chain [40]. Similarly, a deficiency in the overall antigen processing machinery has also been reported. That includes lack of mRNA expression of MHC proteasome genes *LMP-7* and *LMP-2*, as well as MHC-peptide transporter genes, *TAP-1* and *TAP-2*, in human small cell lung carcinoma cells that severely affect the antitumor effector T-cell responses [41]. In addition, tapasin, which is an important member of PLC of MHC1 has been reported to be mutated or generate a deletion splice variant in human cancer cell lines that affects MHC1-peptide transport and surface expression [42] and CTL responses [43] (Fig. 1.2B). Apart from the deficiency in MHC-1 expression, tumors have been reported to lack the expression of costimulatory B7 family (B7-1 and B7-2) molecules. The lack of B7 molecules have been observed in murine-derived cancer cells [44] as well as in primary human cancer cells such as metastatic renal cell carcinoma and nonsmall-cell lung cancers [18,44−46]. The lack of B7 (CD80 and CD86) on tumors can render immunoreactive T cells anergic allowing tumors to escape T-cell-mediated killings [47,48]. Not only has the reduction of B7 molecule observed on tumors, an increase has also been observed in a second B7 costimulatory family, the programmed death ligand (PD-L1). The PD-L1 along with its second member PD-L2 binds to the programmed death 1 (PD1) receptor, which belongs to Ig-V family of costimulatory receptors, the other members of which include CD28, CTLA4, Inducible T-cell co-stimulator (ICOS), and B and T-lymphocyte attenuator (BTLA) [38,49,50]. Interestingly, despite being the members of B7 family, PD-L1 and PD-L2 do not bind to the CD28 or CTLA-4 or ICOS.

Both PD-L1 and PD-L2 are expressed in various human tissues. However, PD-L1 compared to PD-L2 shows greater distribution and expression on tumor tissues [50]. The enhanced PD-L1 expression has

been reported in several different human cancers such as ovarian, lung, colon carcinoma, and melanoma [51,52]. The enhanced expression of PD-L1 on tumors engages T-cell coinhibitory PD1 receptors present on activated antigen-specific T cells that lead to the attenuation of T-cell receptor signaling and antitumor immune responses [48,53] (Fig. 1.2B). The PD1 expression on antigen-specific T cells are initially low that however changes when T cells receive antigenic stimulations. With the persistent activation of T cells, the PD1 expression increases dramatically. PD1 functions as an inhibitory checkpoint receptor molecule. PD1 plays a crucial role in avoiding autoimmune responses that may generate due to strong activation of antigen-specific T cells during antitumor or antiviral responses. In addition, PD1 also plays a predominant role in peripheral tolerance. Interestingly, CD28 cytoplasmic tail contains YxxM signature motif that are phosphorylated by the Src family protein tyrosine kinases p56[lck] and p59[fyn] [54]. The cytoplasmic tail of PD1 receptor contains immunoreceptor tyrosine-based inhibitory motif [(ITIM) VDYGEL] [55,56] and immunoreceptor tyrosine-based switch motif [(ITSM) TEYSEV] [56,57]. The two tyrosine residues are present within the cytoplasmic tail: one in the membrane proximal ITIM and second one in the distal ITSM. These motifs upon engagement with PD-L1 positive tumors undergo tyrosine phosphorylation, and recruit SH2 domain-containing tyrosine phosphatases SHP1 and SHP2. The SHP2 recruitment has been reported to dephosphorylate CD3ζ chain leading to the inhibition of TCR signaling [58]. However, more recently PD1-associated SHP2 have also been shown to dephosphorylate phospho-CD28 [59]. The PD1 has also been reported to lead to inhibition of CD28 costimulatory PI3K/AKT signaling pathway. PD1 ligation inhibits CD28-mediated PI3K kinase activation in a manner that is depended on ITSM [60] (Fig. 1.2B). The SHP1 also gets recruited to the PD1 cytoplasmic tails, its function, however, remains unknown.

Immune Escape Through T-Cell Exhaustion
T-cell exhaustion represents another major immune escape mechanism observed in the immunoreactive cancers and chronic viral infections. Exhaustion of antigen-specific T cells is an acquired state of differentiation presented with altered metabolic and epigenetic phenotype. Exhaustion develops in chronic viral infections such as HIV, HCV, and HBV and also in response to immune reactive cancers such as ovarian cancer, rhabdomyosarcoma, and melanoma that are known to express tumor-specific antigens including the

cancer-germline genes such as *SSX* family (in synovial sarcoma), melanoma antigen *(MAGE) A, B or C* families, and *LAGE* families [61–66]. Exhaustion is initiated with the persistent delivery of signal $1 + 2$ (MHC/TCR + B7/CD28) and maintained by the checkpoint PD1/PDL1 signaling, epigenetic reprogramming such as DNA and histone methylation, and enhanced expression of transcription factors such as YY1, IRF4, NFAT (Balkhi et al., review submitted for publication). The inhibitory PD1/PDL1 signaling is essential to control the proliferation of persistently activated antigen-specific T cells to avoid autoimmune responses. Accordingly, exhausted T cells consistently express markers associated with T-cell activation but have lost the capacity to proliferate and evoking effector responses. One of the distinctive characteristics of exhausted T cells is that they can regain effector functions especially their killing functions against antigenic targets with the antibody-mediated blockade of immune checkpoint receptors (PD1, LAG3, TIM3) as well as noncheckpoint-based therapeutic interventions [67].

Tolerance as a Major Immune Escape Mechanism

The immunosurveillance refers to the power of innate and adaptive immune system to eradicate cancerous growth. The cytolytic T cells and natural killer cells can physically eliminate cancer cells during immunosurveillance. In addition to effector cells, effector cytokines and effector molecules are crucial for the elimination of cancers. Gene targeting studies in mice have demonstrated conclusively that lack of effector molecules such as IFNγ, perforins, TNF-related apoptosis-inducing ligand, or defective mutant Fas Ligand (FasL or CD95L) are crucial for the suppression of cancerous growth [68]. According to the hypothesis of immunosurveillance proposed by Burnet [69], cancers that grow successfully have lost immunogenicity and, thus, escaped immunosurveillance. However, with the recent success of immunotherapy drugs especially checkpoint receptor blockade (CRB) inhibitory antibodies, it has become possible to rejuvenate destructive immune responses against advanced stage cancers, indicating that growth of such cancers cannot be due to the loss of immunogenicity but due to the immune dysfunction that compromised immunosurveillance. The virally induced cancers (e.g., HPV, Epstein–Bar virus), and cancers known to express neoantigens or cancer germline genes (e.g., melanoma and ovarian cancers) are more likely to be eradicated during immunosurveillance or respond positively to the immunotherapy treatments. Such cancers are, therefore,

less likely to have lost the immunogenicity [70,71]. However, the spontaneous cancers that are not known to express neoantigens or cancer germline genes or lack harboring significant deleterious mutations such as gene rearrangements and large insertions but rather present with gene amplifications, small in frame insertions and deletions may be insufficient to produce immunogenic tumor antigens (e.g., breast cancer, colorectal cancers, etc.). Therefore, these cancers are more likely to escape immunosurveillance due to the process of natural selection of "tumor variants with low immunogenicity." The low immunogenicity may still be an underlying mechanism of immune escape despite the driver and passenger mutations within the cancer cells conferring growth advantage and imposing their own natural selection [72]. Overall, low immunogenicity' eventually generates T-cell tolerance, and such low immunogenic cancers are unlikely to benefit from CRB inhibitory drugs and may appear inherently nonimmunogenic [73,74]. However, most of the sporadic cancer mouse models and human tumors regardless of the number and type of mutations in their genome are known to have T-cell infiltration, and some even generate antibody and effector T-cell responses. Even recent data have corroborated that cancers especially colorectal carcinoma with T-cell infiltration are likely to have better prognosis and more likely to respond to the therapy [75]. However, association of T cell infiltrates and better prognosis in cancer is controversial, as conflicting data exist with respect to the colorectal cancers. Colorectal cancer is an important model for our understanding of relationship between cancer, TIL infiltration, and better prognosis. A study by Laghi L et al. demonstrated that CD3 (TIL) infiltration into stage III colorectal cancer cannot be an independent predictor of clinical outcome [76]. How to explain these conflicting data? First, it remains unclear at what stage cancers especially in patients not undergoing any active anticancer treatment might have been more immunogenic to have attracted immune cell infiltration. Second, why tumors would lose immunogenicity or undergo antigen escape in the absence of "selection pressure" that may be imposed by anticancer treatments such as chemo- and radiation- therapy or CAR immunotherapy. A likely explanation could be that T-cell infiltration including the presence of immature myeloid cells, suppressor cytokines, and other factors seen in advanced stage tumors, and also reported in sporadic tumor mouse model must be seen as an antigen-specific tolerogenic response rather an immunogenic response [77].

Loss of Tumor Immunogenicity

The loss of tumor immunogenicity may occur due to the generation of weakly immunogenic tumor antigen variants and due to the "antigen escape". The process of antigen escape came into light recently in the CAR immunotherapy clinical trials. CARs designed to target CD19 expressing B-cell malignancies become ineffective (lose immunogenicity) due to loss of CD19 target antigen on cancer cells, instead new clone of B-cell cancers were formed that were CD19 negative [78]. Data obtained with sporadic cancer mouse models, and in human patients with monoclonal gammopathy suggest that at noninvasive premalignant latent stage, tumors can induce strong adaptive immune responses [23,79]. However, with the progressively growing tumors, such responses may be lost [77,79]. It remains unclear if the loss of immunogenicity and tolerance induction, as seen in advanced stage multiple myeloma in humans that progresses from premalignant monoclonal gammopathy [79], occurs due to the tumors losing immunogenicity or due to tolerance induction in T cells reacting to less immunogenic tumor antigen variants arising in progressively growing tumors [80,81]. The rise of less immunogenic tumor antigen variants in advanced stage cancers have also been demonstrated in immunocompetent murine sporadic epithelial carcinoma model [82]. The latter point may seem contradictory that tumors at advanced stage become less immunogenic due to rise of less immunogenic tumor antigen variants. In contrast, it may be expected that with the advanced stage tumors, growth of more immunogenic tumor antigen variants may occur as with the "age of tumors" more mutagenic events are likely to accumulate. The evidences of less immunogenic antigen variants arising in progressively growing cancers have come mostly from the sporadic cancer mouse models [83]. In such mouse models, cancer progression can be rapid whereas human spontaneous cancers may take several years to grow, therefore, the mouse data must be interpreted with caution [80].

Immune Tolerance: A Natural Checkpoint Protecting Cancers From Immune Recognition and Eradication

Immune tolerance is a crucial arm of adaptive immunity that develops in thymus early in the life of an individual. Tolerance allows T cells to recognize nonself-antigens as immunogenic while self-antigens as nonimmunogenic. That helps to avoid autoimmune responses during immunosurveillance.

T cells learn to become tolerant to self-antigens during their development in thymus. The committed lymphocyte progenitors that develop from hematopoietic stem cells in the bone marrow migrate to thymus where T-cell progenitors (thymocytes) differentiate into double positive (DP; TCR^+CD4^+ $CD8^+$) thymocytes after transitioning from successive double negative T-cell development stages (DN1-DN4; $TCR^-CD4^-CD8^-$) [84]. The DP T cells scan the cortical thymic epithelial cells (cTEC). The cTEC processes endogenous proteins (self-antigens) to load on MHC class I molecules utilizing proteasome machinery containing a catalytic subunit unique to cTEC known as β5t (thymoproteasome) [85,86]. Similarly, cTEC also process endogenous proteins to load on MHC class II molecule that involves lysosomal macroautophagy of cytoplasmic proteins followed by processing through Cathepsin L and thymus-specific serine protease. These along with the cortical conventional dendritic cells (cDCs) present self-antigens to the DP thymocytes to initiate the positive selection process. It is obvious that the cTEC plays a vital role in the positive selection process due to its unique location and special antigen-processing machinery [87]. The DP thymocytes that react self-antigens with low-affinity, that is, initiating optimal TCR signaling are positively selected [88] to become lineage committed to differentiate into SP ($CD4^+$ and $CD8^+$) T cells in which T-cell receptor (αβTCR) and coreceptor signaling strength play a crucial role [84]. The negative selection of DP thymocytes in mice occur in thymic cortex [89], whereas second wave of negative selection of SP T cells occur in medulla [90]. In negative selection, TCRs that react strongly with the self-peptides, that is, initiating excessive TCR signaling are deleted through apoptosis. As shown by Stritesky et al. in murine system, 75% of DP T cells die in the cortex, whereas 25% that die in the medulla are SP T cells [90]. Overall, negative selection efficiently deletes self-antigen reactive (autoreactive) T cells that otherwise could lead to damaging autoimmune responses. Apart from the negative selection, 90% of DP T cells die of neglect, that is, due to lack of positive selection in the thymic cortex as they fail to engage with self-peptide loaded MHCs of thymic epithelial cells and thymic APCs [86]. Eventually, only a small fraction of T cells are positively selected to exit the thymus.

The lineage committed SP ($CD4^+$ or $CD8^+$) T cells in the thymic medulla scan medullary thymic epithelial cells (mTEC) and medullary antigen-presenting cells (mAPCs) that include among others the resident and migratory conventional dendritic cells (cDCs), plasmatoid dendritic cells (pDCs), and B cells. Therefore, in the medulla SP T cells may be exposed to peripheral self-antigens through immigrating pDCs. The lineage committed SP T cells that have initiated intermediate level of TCR signaling upon engagement with self-peptide-loaded MHC class I and MHC class II differentiate into $CD8^+$ and $CD4^+$ T cells, respectively [84]. Finally, T cells after having received the education to be tolerant to self-antigens exit thymic medulla and enter into blood circulation to be transported to tissues and secondary lymphoid organs to join peripheral T-cell pool to function in adaptive T-cell responses. However, some T cells can escape death by neglect as well as negative selection in the thymus [91]. In addition, not all self-reactive TCRs can be eliminated in the thymus because not all self-antigens exist in the thymus. The T cells in the periphery encounter new self-antigens. Therefore, peripheral tolerance mechanism exist that ensures self-reactive T cells are eliminated in the periphery. In peripheral tolerance the high affinity self-reactive T cells and those TCRs that might have escaped negative selection become deleted through Fas-FasL and Bim-mediated apoptosis or are rendered anergic. Therefore, these mechanisms render peripheral T-cell pool unlikely to be autoreactive, and fully functional against nonself-antigens [88,92,93]. How exactly T cells distinguish optimal affinity versus high affinity self-antigens is not completely understood. However, the role of Ca^{2+} influx and extracellular signal-regulated kinase (ERK) activity in vivo appears crucial for both negative and positive selection. For example, in the negative selection, rapid ERK activation occurs that sustains for a brief duration (peak at 2 minutes) triggering cell death. In contrast, in positive selection, ERK activation occurs at lower kinetics that sustains for longer duration (96 hours) [94]. Another protein reported to be crucial for the positive and negative selection in the thymus is thymocyte-expressed molecule involved in selection (Themis). Mice deficient in Themis exhibit defects both in positive and negative selection. Experimental data suggest that TCR signaling triggers phosphorylation of Themis and phosphorylated Themis appears to regulate calcium influx and ERK kinase phosphorylation [95].

From the above description about the generation of T-cell tolerance to self-peptides, it is not unconceivable to imagine that because most tumors express antigens that are self-antigens, our immune system simply ignores the tumor growth. Thus, tolerance acts as a natural barrier protecting tumors. The self-antigens that are mostly expressed by the tumors are termed as tumor-associated antigens (TAA), numerous examples of which exist including Her2/neu, CEA, CD19, CD22, and mucin. However, apart from the tumor-associated self-antigens, there are antigens that are expressed uniquely in tumors. These are termed as tumor-specific antigens (TSA). The example of tumor-specific antigens is the cancer germline genes (CCG) [66,96]. The cancer germline genes are mostly expressed in male reproductive tissues such as spermatogonia or in the embryonic cells. However, in cancer, these embryonic or cancer germline genes can get reexpressed. An example of cancer germline genes include *MAGE*, *LAGE* family genes, which are reexpressed in melanoma [66]. Because the T cells during their development in thymus are not exposed to the cancer germline genes. T cells, therefore, are able to react with the tumors expressing cancer germline genes and eliminate them [97]. Melanoma, therefore, is one of the rare cancers that attract T cells. Another class of cancer-specific antigens from the family of cancer germline genes include *SSX* family, which is expressed in sarcoma [98]. Almost 70 families comprising 140 individual genes have been associated with the cancer germline family [99]. The reason why cancer germline genes are recognized by the T cells as nonself is because spermatogonia tissues in humans does not express MHC-1 molecules. Therefore, T cells during the generation of peripheral tolerance may not get exposed to these antigens and as such cannot recognize them as self-antigens. The later point was proven in a study in which transgenic mice were generated with cancer germline genes and T cells isolated from such mice does not evoke immune responses indicating that T cells become tolerant to such antigens and recognize them as self-antigens [97].

Unfortunately, most cancers express tumor-associated antigens that are self-antigens, naturally T cells recognize them as self-antigens. Therefore, as expected, no antitumor immune response could be generated providing such tumors an efficient means to escape. The problem encountering immunotherapy field is the tolerance imposed by the tumor-associated antigens. In contrast, the TSAs because of their capacity to attract T cells, and with simple immunotherapeutic interventions such as adoptive T-cell transfer plus infusions of high doses of IL2 can elicit immunoreactivity and successful eradication of cancers as demonstrated for immunogenic melanoma and sarcoma [71,100–105]. Therefore, that provides strong rationale to design therapeutics to force T cells to react with the less immunogenic cancers expressing tumor associated self-antigens (TAAs). The pitfall of reactivity and damage to healthy tissues may be inevitable for such therapies. CAR therapy is the therapeutic intervention that through the expression of chimeric receptor antibody forces T cells to react with the tumor-associated antigens bypassing the lack of MHC presentation or reduced MHC and costimulatory molecules, as well as barriers imposed by the tolerance to self-antigens. These

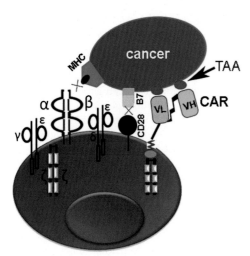

FIG. 1.3 Schematic illustration conceptualizing how chimeric antigen receptors (CARs) can help T cells to recognize tumor-associated antigens by successfully overcoming the barriers imposed by the immune escape mechanisms, for example, dysregulated antigen processing and presentation as well as reduced costimulatory molecule expression.

underlying concepts behind designing CARs works elegantly, and today CAR therapy is one of the most promising therapy being developed to eradicate cancers utilizing autologous T cells because T cells are biologically programmed to target tumors, and T cells have power to physically eradicate cancer cells through synthesis and secretion of granzymes, perforins, and cytokines. Conferring the antibody-directed specificity on T cells allows T cells to eradicate cancer cells by bypassing not only tolerance but also other immune escape mechanisms developed by tumors such as reduced costimulatory molecules or defective antigen processing and presentations (Fig. 1.3). In Chapter 2, we will learn about the components of CARs and how CARs are generated to target tumors.

REFERENCES

[1] Littman RJ. The plague of Athens: epidemiology and paleopathology. Mt Sinai J Med 2009;76:456–67.

[2] Hoption Cann SA, van Netten JP, van Netten C. Dr William Coley and tumour regression: a place in history or in the future. Postgrad Med J 2003;79:672–80.

[3] Coley WB. The treatment of inoperable sarcoma by bacterial toxins (the mixed toxins of the Streptococcus erysipelas and the Bacillus prodigiosus). Proc R Soc Med 1910;3:1–48.

[4] Coley WB. The treatment of malignant tumors by repeated inoculations of erysipelas. With a report of ten original cases. 1893. Clin Orthop Relat Res 1991:3–11.

[5] Nauts HC, Fowler GA, Bogatko FH. A review of the influence of bacterial infection and of bacterial products (Coley's toxins) on malignant tumors in man; a critical analysis of 30 inoperable cases treated by Coley's mixed toxins, in which diagnosis was confirmed by microscopic examination selected for special study. Acta Med Scand Suppl 1953;276:1–103.

[6] Gross G, Gorochov G, Waks T, Eshhar Z. Generation of effector T cells expressing chimeric T cell receptor with antibody type-specificity. Transplant Proc 1989;21:127–30.

[7] Gross G, Waks T, Eshhar Z. Expression of immunoglobulin-T-cell receptor chimeric molecules as functional receptors with antibody-type specificity. Proc Natl Acad Sci U S A 1989;86:10024–8.

[8] Abate-Daga D, Davila ML. CAR models: next-generation CAR modifications for enhanced T-cell function. Mol Ther Oncolytics 2016;3:16014.

[9] Rosenberg SA, Packard BS, Aebersold PM, Solomon D, Topalian SL, Toy ST, et al. Use of tumor-infiltrating lymphocytes and interleukin-2 in the immunotherapy of patients with metastatic melanoma. A preliminary report. N Engl J Med 1988;319:1676–80.

[10] Rosenberg SA, Yang JC, Sherry RM, Kammula US, Hughes MS, Phan GQ, et al. Durable complete responses in heavily pretreated patients with metastatic melanoma using T-cell transfer immunotherapy. Clin Cancer Res 2011;17:4550–7.

[11] Dudley ME. Adoptive cell therapy for patients with melanoma. J Cancer 2011;2:360–2.

[12] Restifo NP, Dudley ME, Rosenberg SA. Adoptive immunotherapy for cancer: harnessing the T cell response. Nat Rev Immunol 2012;12:269–81.

[13] Robbins PF, Lu YC, El-Gamil M, Li YF, Gross C, Gartner J, et al. Mining exomic sequencing data to identify mutated antigens recognized by adoptively transferred tumor-reactive T cells. Nat Med 2013;19:747–52.

[14] Lim WA, June CH. The principles of engineering immune cells to treat cancer. Cell 2017;168:724–40.

[15] Rosenberg SA, Tran E, Robbins PF. T-cell transfer therapy targeting mutant KRAS. N Engl J Med 2017;376:e11.

[16] Tran E, Robbins PF, Rosenberg SA. 'Final common pathway' of human cancer immunotherapy: targeting random somatic mutations. Nat Immunol 2017;18:255–62.

[17] Robbins PF, El-Gamil M, Li YF, Kawakami Y, Loftus D, Appella E, et al. A mutated beta-catenin gene encodes a melanoma-specific antigen recognized by tumor infiltrating lymphocytes. J Exp Med 1996;183:1185–92.

[18] Driessens G, Kline J, Gajewski TF. Costimulatory and coinhibitory receptors in anti-tumor immunity. Immunol Rev 2009;229:126–44.

[19] Galon J, Costes A, Sanchez-Cabo F, Kirilovsky A, Mlecnik B, Lagorce-Pages C, et al. Type, density, and location of immune cells within human colorectal tumors predict clinical outcome. Science 2006;313:1960–4.

[20] Hwang WT, Adams SF, Tahirovic E, Hagemann IS, Coukos G. Prognostic significance of tumor-infiltrating T cells in ovarian cancer: a meta-analysis. Gynecol Oncol 2012;124:192—8.

[21] Mahmoud SM, Paish EC, Powe DG, Macmillan RD, Grainge MJ, Lee AH, et al. Tumor-infiltrating CD8$^+$ lymphocytes predict clinical outcome in breast cancer. J Clin Oncol 2011;29:1949—55.

[22] Nguyen LT, Elford AR, Murakami K, Garza KM, Schoenberger SP, Odermatt B, et al. Tumor growth enhances cross-presentation leading to limited T cell activation without tolerance. J Exp Med 2002;195:423—35.

[23] Willimsky G, Czeh M, Loddenkemper C, Gellermann J, Schmidt K, Wust P, et al. Immunogenicity of premalignant lesions is the primary cause of general cytotoxic T lymphocyte unresponsiveness. J Exp Med 2008;205: 1687—700.

[24] Lennerz V, Fatho M, Gentilini C, Frye RA, Lifke A, Ferel D, et al. The response of autologous T cells to a human melanoma is dominated by mutated neoantigens. Proc Natl Acad Sci U S A 2005;102:16013—8.

[25] Fearon ER, Vogelstein B. A genetic model for colorectal tumorigenesis. Cell 1990;61:759—67.

[26] Ganusov VV, De Boer RJ. Do most lymphocytes in humans really reside in the gut? Trends Immunol 2007;28:514—8.

[27] Blum JS, Wearsch PA, Cresswell P. Pathways of antigen processing. Annu Rev Immunol 2013;31:443—73.

[28] Turcotte S, Rosenberg SA. Immunotherapy for metastatic solid cancers. Adv Surg 2011;45:341—60.

[29] Smith-Garvin JE, Koretzky GA, Jordan MS. T cell activation. Annu Rev Immunol 2009;27:591—619.

[30] Neefjes J, Jongsma ML, Paul P, Bakke O. Towards a systems understanding of MHC class I and MHC class II antigen presentation. Nat Rev Immunol 2011;11: 823—36.

[31] Shepherd JC, Schumacher TN, Ashton-Rickardt PG, Imaeda S, Ploegh HL, Janeway Jr CA, et al. TAP1-dependent peptide translocation in vitro is ATP dependent and peptide selective. Cell 1993;74:577—84.

[32] Hulpke S, Tampe R. The MHC I loading complex: a multitasking machinery in adaptive immunity. Trends Biochem Sci 2013;38:412—20.

[33] Ortmann B, Copeman J, Lehner PJ, Sadasivan B, Herberg JA, Grandea AG, et al. A critical role for tapasin in the assembly and function of multimeric MHC class I-TAP complexes. Science 1997;277:1306—9.

[34] Blees A, Januliene D, Hofmann T, Koller N, Schmidt C, Trowitzsch S, et al. Structure of the human MHC-I peptide-loading complex. Nature 2017;551:525—8.

[35] Hussain A, Mohammad DK, Gustafsson MO, Uslu M, Hamasy A, Nore BF, et al. Signaling of the ITK (interleukin 2-inducible T cell kinase)-SYK (spleen tyrosine kinase) fusion kinase is dependent on adapter SLP-76 and on the adapter function of the kinases SYK and ZAP70. J Biol Chem 2013;288:7338—50.

[36] Wang H, Kadlecek TA, Au-Yeung BB, Goodfellow HE, Hsu LY, Freedman TS, et al. ZAP-70: an essential kinase in T-cell signaling. Cold Spring Harb Perspect Biol 2010; 2:a002279.

[37] Lenschow DJ, Walunas TL, Bluestone JA. CD28/B7 system of T cell costimulation. Annu Rev Immunol 1996; 14:233—58.

[38] Boomer JS, Green JM. An enigmatic tail of CD28 signaling. Cold Spring Harb Perspect Biol 2010;2: a002436.

[39] Elliott BE, Carlow DA, Rodricks AM, Wade A. Perspectives on the role of MHC antigens in normal and malignant cell development. Adv Cancer Res 1989;53: 181—245.

[40] D'Urso CM, Wang ZG, Cao Y, Tatake R, Zeff RA, Ferrone S. Lack of HLA class I antigen expression by cultured melanoma cells FO-1 due to a defect in B2m gene expression. J Clin Invest 1991;87:284—92.

[41] Restifo NP, Esquivel F, Kawakami Y, Yewdell JW, Mule JJ, Rosenberg SA, et al. Identification of human cancers deficient in antigen processing. J Exp Med 1993;177:265—72.

[42] Belicha-Villanueva A, Golding M, McEvoy S, Sarvaiya N, Cresswell P, Gollnick SO, et al. Identification of an alternate splice form of tapasin in human melanoma. Hum Immunol 2010;71:1018—26.

[43] Shionoya Y, Kanaseki T, Miyamoto S, Tokita S, Hongo A, Kikuchi Y, et al. Loss of tapasin in human lung and colon cancer cells and escape from tumor-associated antigen-specific CTL recognition. OncoImmunology 2017;6:e1274476.

[44] Chen L, McGowan P, Ashe S, Johnston J, Li Y, Hellstrom I, et al. Tumor immunogenicity determines the effect of B7 costimulation on T cell-mediated tumor immunity. J Exp Med 1994;179:523—32.

[45] Antonia SJ, Seigne J, Diaz J, Muro-Cacho C, Extermann M, Farmelo MJ, et al. Phase I trial of a B7-1 (CD80) gene modified autologous tumor cell vaccine in combination with systemic interleukin-2 in patients with metastatic renal cell carcinoma. J Urol 2002;167: 1995—2000.

[46] Raez LE, Cassileth PA, Schlesselman JJ, Sridhar K, Padmanabhan S, Fisher EZ, et al. Allogeneic vaccination with a B7.1 HLA-A gene-modified adenocarcinoma cell line in patients with advanced non-small-cell lung cancer. J Clin Oncol 2004;22:2800—7.

[47] Zou W, Chen L. Inhibitory B7-family molecules in the tumour microenvironment. Nat Rev Immunol 2008;8: 467—77.

[48] Crespo J, Sun H, Welling TH, Tian Z, Zou W. T cell anergy, exhaustion, senescence, and stemness in the tumor microenvironment. Curr Opin Immunol 2013;25: 214—21.

[49] Freeman GJ, Long AJ, Iwai Y, Bourque K, Chernova T, Nishimura H, et al. Engagement of the PD-1 immunoinhibitory receptor by a novel B7 family member leads to negative regulation of lymphocyte activation. J Exp Med 2000;192:1027—34.

[50] Latchman Y, Wood CR, Chernova T, Chaudhary D, Borde M, Chernova I, et al. PD-L2 is a second ligand

for PD-1 and inhibits T cell activation. Nat Immunol 2001;2:261−8.

[51] Bardhan K, Anagnostou T, Boussiotis VA. The PD1:PD-L1/2 pathway from discovery to clinical implementation. Front Immunol 2016;7:550.

[52] Dong H, Strome SE, Salomao DR, Tamura H, Hirano F, Flies DB, et al. Tumor-associated B7-H1 promotes T-cell apoptosis: a potential mechanism of immune evasion. Nat Med 2002;8:793−800.

[53] Curiel TJ, Wei S, Dong H, Alvarez X, Cheng P, Mottram P, et al. Blockade of B7-H1 improves myeloid dendritic cell-mediated antitumor immunity. Nat Med 2003;9:562−7.

[54] Rudd CE, Schneider H. Unifying concepts in CD28, ICOS and CTLA4 co-receptor signalling. Nat Rev Immunol 2003;3:544−56.

[55] Ishida Y, Agata Y, Shibahara K, Honjo T. Induced expression of PD-1, a novel member of the immunoglobulin gene superfamily, upon programmed cell death. EMBO J 1992;11:3887−95.

[56] Krueger J, Rudd CE. Two strings in one bow: PD-1 negatively regulates via Co-receptor CD28 on T cells. Immunity 2017;46:529−31.

[57] Leibson PJ. The regulation of lymphocyte activation by inhibitory receptors. Curr Opin Immunol 2004;16: 328−36.

[58] Salmond RJ, Alexander DR. SHP2 forecast for the immune system: fog gradually clearing. Trends Immunol 2006;27:154−60.

[59] Hui E, Cheung J, Zhu J, Su X, Taylor MJ, Wallweber HA, et al. T cell costimulatory receptor CD28 is a primary target for PD-1-mediated inhibition. Science 2017;355: 1428−33.

[60] Parry RV, Chemnitz JM, Frauwirth KA, Lanfranco AR, Braunstein I, Kobayashi SV, et al. CTLA-4 and PD-1 receptors inhibit T-cell activation by distinct mechanisms. Mol Cell Biol 2005;25:9543−53.

[61] Sen DR, Kaminski J, Barnitz RA, Kurachi M, Gerdemann U, Yates KB, et al. The epigenetic landscape of T cell exhaustion. Science 2016;354:1165−9.

[62] Scott-Browne JP, Lopez-Moyado IF, Trifari S, Wong V, Chavez L, Rao A, et al. Dynamic changes in chromatin accessibility occur in CD8(+) T cells responding to viral infection. Immunity 2016;45:1327−40.

[63] Pauken KE, Sammons MA, Odorizzi PM, Manne S, Godec J, Khan O, et al. Epigenetic stability of exhausted T cells limits durability of reinvigoration by PD-1 blockade. Science 2016;354:1160−5.

[64] Hashimoto M, Kamphorst AO, Im SJ, Kissick HT, Pillai RN, Ramalingam SS, et al. CD8 T cell exhaustion in chronic infection and cancer: opportunities for interventions. Annu Rev Immunol 2018;69:301−18.

[65] Balkhi MY, Ma Q, Ahmad S, Junghans RP. T cell exhaustion and Interleukin 2 downregulation. Cytokine 2015; 71:339−47.

[66] van der Bruggen P, Traversari C, Chomez P, Lurquin C, De Plaen E, Van den Eynde B, et al. A gene encoding an antigen recognized by cytolytic T lymphocytes on a human melanoma. Science 1991;254:1643−7.

[67] Wherry EJ. T cell exhaustion. Nat Immunol 2011;12: 492−9.

[68] Swann JB, Smyth MJ. Immune surveillance of tumors. J Clin Invest 2007;117:1137−46.

[69] Burnet M. Immunological factors in the process of carcinogenesis. Br Med Bull 1964;20:154−8.

[70] Klein G, Klein E. Immune surveillance against virus-induced tumors and nonrejectability of spontaneous tumors: contrasting consequences of host versus tumor evolution. Proc Natl Acad Sci U S A 1977;74:2121−5.

[71] Rosenberg SA, Mule JJ, Spiess PJ, Reichert CM, Schwarz SL. Regression of established pulmonary metastases and subcutaneous tumor mediated by the systemic administration of high-dose recombinant interleukin 2. J Exp Med 1985;161:1169−88.

[72] Stratton MR, Campbell PJ, Futreal PA. The cancer genome. Nature 2009;458:719−24.

[73] Stutman O. Spontaneous tumors in nude mice: effect of the viable yellow gene. Exp Cell Biol 1979;47:129−35.

[74] Stutman O. Tumor development after 3-methylcholanthrene in immunologically deficient athymic-nude mice. Science 1974;183:534−6.

[75] Jochems C, Schlom J. Tumor-infiltrating immune cells and prognosis: the potential link between conventional cancer therapy and immunity. Exp Biol Med 2011;236:567−79.

[76] Laghi L, Bianchi P, Miranda E, Balladore E, Pacetti V, Grizzi F, et al. CD3+ cells at the invasive margin of deeply invading (pT3-T4) colorectal cancer and risk of post-surgical metastasis: a longitudinal study. Lancet Oncol 2009;10:877−84.

[77] Willimsky G, Blankenstein T. Sporadic immunogenic tumours avoid destruction by inducing T-cell tolerance. Nature 2005;437:141−6.

[78] Zah E, Lin MY, Silva-Benedict A, Jensen MC, Chen YY. T cells expressing CD19/CD20 bi-specific chimeric antigen receptors prevent antigen escape by malignant B cells. Cancer Immunol Res 2016.

[79] Dhodapkar MV, Krasovsky J, Osman K, Geller MD. Vigorous premalignancy-specific effector T cell response in the bone marrow of patients with monoclonal gammopathy. J Exp Med 2003;198:1753−7.

[80] Khong HT, Restifo NP. Natural selection of tumor variants in the generation of "tumor escape" phenotypes. Nat Immunol 2002;3:999−1005.

[81] Schreiber H, Wu TH, Nachman J, Kast WM. Immunodominance and tumor escape. Semin Cancer Biol 2002;12: 25−31.

[82] Shankaran V, Ikeda H, Bruce AT, White JM, Swanson PE, Old LJ, et al. IFNgamma and lymphocytes prevent primary tumour development and shape tumour immunogenicity. Nature 2001;410:1107−11.

[83] Jonkers J, Berns A. Conditional mouse models of sporadic cancer. Nat Rev Cancer 2002;2:251−65.

[84] Germain RN. T-cell development and the CD4-CD8 lineage decision. Nat Rev Immunol 2002;2:309−22.

[85] Florea BI, Verdoes M, Li N, van der Linden WA, Geurink PP, van den Elst H, et al. Activity-based profiling reveals reactivity of the murine thymoproteasome-specific subunit beta5t. Chem Biol 2010;17:795−801.

[86] Klein L, Kyewski B, Allen PM, Hogquist KA. Positive and negative selection of the T cell repertoire: what thymocytes see (and don't see). Nat Rev Immunol 2014;14:377−91.

[87] Klein L, Hinterberger M, Wirnsberger G, Kyewski B. Antigen presentation in the thymus for positive selection and central tolerance induction. Nat Rev Immunol 2009;9:833−44.

[88] Xing Y, Hogquist KA. T-cell tolerance: central and peripheral. Cold Spring Harb Perspect Biol 2012;4.

[89] Surh CD, Sprent J. T-cell apoptosis detected in situ during positive and negative selection in the thymus. Nature 1994;372:100−3.

[90] Stritesky GL, Xing Y, Erickson JR, Kalekar LA, Wang X, Mueller DL, et al. Murine thymic selection quantified using a unique method to capture deleted T cells. Proc Natl Acad Sci U S A 2013;110:4679−84.

[91] Fink PJ, McMahan CJ. Lymphocytes rearrange, edit and revise their antigen receptors to be useful yet safe. Immunol Today 2000;21:561−6.

[92] Kroemer G, Martinez C. Mechanisms of self tolerance. Immunol Today 1992;13:401−4.

[93] Miller JF, Basten A. Mechanisms of tolerance to self. Curr Opin Immunol 1996;8:815−21.

[94] McNeil LK, Starr TK, Hogquist KA. A requirement for sustained ERK signaling during thymocyte positive selection in vivo. Proc Natl Acad Sci U S A 2005;102:13574−9.

[95] Fu G, Vallee S, Rybakin V, McGuire MV, Ampudia J, Brockmeyer C, et al. Themis controls thymocyte selection through regulation of T cell antigen receptor-mediated signaling. Nat Immunol 2009;10:848−56.

[96] van den Brink EN, Bril WS, Turenhout EA, Zuurveld M, Bovenschen N, Peters M, et al. Two classes of germline genes both derived from the V(H)1 family direct the formation of human antibodies that recognize distinct antigenic sites in the C2 domain of factor VIII. Blood 2002;99:2828−34.

[97] Blankenstein T, Coulie PG, Gilboa E, Jaffee EM. The determinants of tumour immunogenicity. Nat Rev Cancer 2012;12:307−13.

[98] Smith HA, McNeel DG. The SSX family of cancer-testis antigens as target proteins for tumor therapy. Clin Dev Immunol 2010;2010:150591.

[99] Ghafouri-Fard S, Modarressi MH. Cancer-testis antigens: potential targets for cancer immunotherapy. Arch Iran Med 2009;12:395−404.

[100] Rosenberg SA, Lotze MT, Muul LM, Leitman S, Chang AE, Ettinghausen SE, et al. Observations on the systemic administration of autologous lymphokine-activated killer cells and recombinant interleukin-2 to patients with metastatic cancer. N Engl J Med 1985;313:1485−92.

[101] Wherry EJ, Blattman JN, Murali-Krishna K, van der Most R, Ahmed R. Viral persistence alters CD8 T-cell immunodominance and tissue distribution and results in distinct stages of functional impairment. J Virol 2003;77:4911−27.

[102] Emtage PC, Lo AS, Gomes EM, Liu DL, Gonzalo-Daganzo RM, Junghans RP. Second-generation anti-carcinoembryonic antigen designer T cells resist activation-induced cell death, proliferate on tumor contact, secrete cytokines, and exhibit superior antitumor activity in vivo: a preclinical evaluation. Clin Cancer Res 2008;14:8112−22.

[103] Lo AS, Ma Q, Liu DL, Junghans RP. Anti-GD3 chimeric sFv-CD28/T-cell receptor zeta designer T cells for treatment of metastatic melanoma and other neuroectodermal tumors. Clin Cancer Res 2010;16:2769−80.

[104] Liao W, Lin JX, Leonard WJ. Interleukin-2 at the crossroads of effector responses, tolerance, and immunotherapy. Immunity 2013;38:13−25.

[105] Zacharakis N, Chinnasamy H, Black M, Xu H, Lu YC, Zheng Z, et al. Immune recognition of somatic mutations leading to complete durable regression in metastatic breast cancer. Nat Med 2018.

CHAPTER 2

Components and Design of Chimeric Antigen Receptors

PROTOTYPICAL DESIGN OF CHIMERIC ANTIGEN RECEPTORS

For CAR-T therapy, the first step involves genetically modifying T-cell receptors with an antigen-binding domain of an *immunoglobulin (Ig)* through advanced gene cloning techniques. The genetically modified T-cell receptors are termed as chimeric antigen receptors (CARs) and T cells having their receptors modified are termed as CAR-T cells. CAR-T cells, therefore, are capable of antibody redirected and MHC-independent target cell killings because such T cells does not depend on antigen presentation for target recognition rather antibody redirects such T cells to access tumor antigens [5–7]. This approach, therefore, apart from providing antibody redirected specificity for antigen recognition combines T cells capacity to lyse tumors. Overall, this approach can help to block immune and antigen escape mechanisms, as well as successfully overcome three main hurdles imposed by the tumors:

(1) Lack of tumor antigen presentation and costimulation. Tumors often reduce expression of MHC class I as well as costimulatory molecules [8–12]. Costimulatory molecules are strongly expressed on antigen presenting cells and may not be even expressed on cancer cells. MHC Class I and costimulatory molecules are crucial for T-cell antigen recognition and delivery of strong intracellular signaling cascade for productive antitumor cytotoxic responses [13]. (2) Anergy [14]. The unmodified tumor-specific T cells become often anergic in tumor environment due to the tumors lacking costimulatory molecules. Therefore, tumor antigen-specific T cells become hyporesponsive and lose ability to produce cytokines compromising their proliferation and tumor-killing activities [15,16]. (3) T-cell tolerance. The unmodified T cells express low-affinity TCRs that are selected to recognize nonself antigens. Most tumors, however, express antigens that are self-antigens, and T cells rarely target those antigens. That allows tumors to escape immunosurveillance [17]. T cells modified with chimeric antibody allow recognizing tumor antigens without relying on optimal low-affinity TCRs. Therefore, CAR T cells can effectively bypass tolerance imposed by self-antigens. A drawback of this approach, however, is that CAR T cells may induce on-target/off-tumor toxicity due to self-antigen reactivity that can trigger autoimmune responses. Moreover, CAR T cells can also lose antigen-specific reactivity in vivo due to antigen escape and may also show lack of in vivo persistence. Intense efforts are being invested to overcome these limitations to make CAR T-cell therapy more potent and safer.

CARs can be designed to target antigens of choice. Primarily, CARs have been designed to target cancers. Nevertheless, several CARs have also been constructed to target viral antigens, but none have been listed to date in human clinical trial database https://clinicaltrials.gov/. CARs are now categorized into first, second, and third generation based on the number of costimulatory molecules incorporated into their design.

The design of various generation of CARs. Chimeric genes are cloned in expression vectors to produce CARs. The vectors commonly employed to clone chimeric genes are retroviral [18] and lentiviral based [19]. However, very recently, a transposon or so-called "sleeping beauty"-based system have also been tested [20,21]. Overall, the retroviral-based vectors that have been extensively tailored to be safer for human use are preferred due to ease of production, control over tropism, that is, to alter infectivity, and better control over CAR expression. These features are important to achieve better antitumor responses in vivo. The advantages and disadvantages of retroviruses have been well established but the transposon-based (SB) system, which is the most advanced nonviral-based vector system, have only recently begun to be evaluated clinically [22–25]. These will be discussed in detail under the section choice of CAR vector systems (Chapter 3).

CAR chimeric genes contain sequences that expresses single-chain variable fragment (scFv) of heavy and light chain of a monoclonal antibody recognizing a specific antigen (Fig. 2.1A). The variable heavy and light chains in scFvs are connected together with a peptide linker

(Fig. 2.1B). In addition to scFv, CARs contain a hinge that is designed to support scFvs, a transmembrane domain, and signaling endodomain that initiate intracellular signaling cascade in response to antigen recognition (Fig. 2.1C).

The first-generation CARs do not contain costimulatory molecules (Fig. 2.2). All CARs including the first, second, and third-generation CARs incorporate a hinge (spacer) that connects scFv with the intracellular signaling domain. The hinge is usually derived from CD8α glycoprotein or IgG constant domains. The CD8α hinge encompasses plasma membrane through its hydrophobic transmembrane domain. Part of the transmembrane domain may contain sequences of costimulatory molecules. Finally, transmembrane domain is fused with the endodomain fusion protein, which is composed of costimulatory molecule(s) fused with the FcεRI γ chain or CD3ε or CD3ζ signaling domains [5,26,27]. The costimulatory molecules usually consist of CD28 or 4-IBB or OX-40 that are fused together with endodomain signaling domain usually derived from CD3ζ sequences (Fig. 2.3). A third-generation CAR incorporates apart from scFv, two costimulatory molecules fused together with CD3ζ endodomain in one-chain single vector (e.g., retroviral vectors) (Fig. 2.4A−C) or two-chain single vector (e.g., retroviral vectors) (Fig. 2.4D−F). A two-chain single vector after cleaving expresses two chains, one will

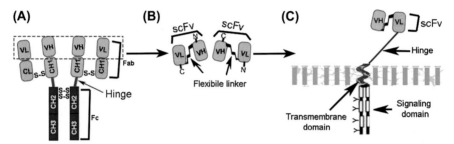

FIG. 2.1 Antibody domain structures and designations commonly applied to refer antibody fragments. **(A)** Full-length antibody comprising typically two heavy and two light chains. Each heavy and light chain possesses variable domains (box) and framework regions that support variable light and variable heavy chain structure. Besides variable domains, a light chain possesses one constant domain region whereas heavy chain can possess multiple typically three constant domains except IgE and IgM that possess a total of four constant domains. **(B)** The structure of a single-chain variable fragment (scFv). A single-chain variable fragment can be constructed from either of the two heavy and two light chains linked through a flexible linker that always connects a light variable chain with variable heavy chain domain. **(C)** Structural organization of a single-chain variable fragment-based chimeric antigen receptors (CARs) when expressed in cells.

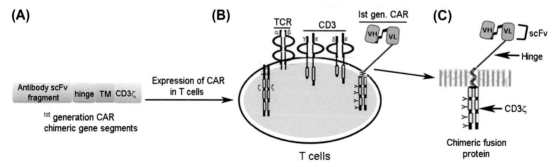

FIG. 2.2 Structural organization of a first-generation CAR. **(A)** Chimeric gene sequence of first-generation CAR encoding scFv, an antigen binding domain that recognizes tumor-associated antigen, a hinge, a transmembrane domain (TM), and a signaling domain, for example, CD3ζ. First-generation CARs do not possess a costimulatory molecule but contains intracellular signaling domain. **(B)** Chimeric first-generation CAR expression in T cells. Chimeric gene sequences are expressed in T cells using various gene transfection methods. The chimeric gene sequence in T cells upon protein translation expresses a fully functional CAR without perturbing endogenous T-cell receptors. **(C)** A magnified view along with various domains of a typical first-generation CAR when expressed in T cells.

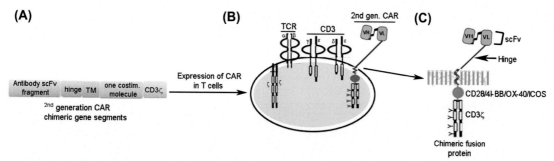

FIG. 2.3 Structural organization of a second-generation CAR. **(A)** Chimeric gene sequence of a second-generation CAR. Second-generation CAR incorporates one costimulatory molecule, typically CD28 or 4I-BB; however, several other costimulatory molecules such as OX40 and ICOS have also been incorporated. **(B)** Chimeric second-generation CAR expression in T cells. Various gene transfection methods can be employed to express plasmids encoding chimeric gene sequences. The chimeric gene sequences in T cells upon protein translation express a fully functional CAR consisting of an ectodomain, a transmembrane domain, and an endogenous costimulatory and signaling domain. The endogenous T-cell receptor remains unperturbed as described in Fig. 2.2. **(C)** A magnified view of a typical second-generation CAR when expressed in T cells.

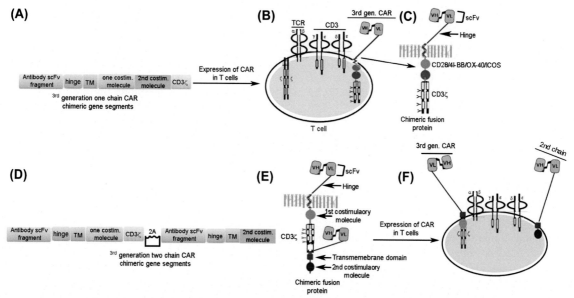

FIG. 2.4 Structural organization of a typical third-generation one chain CAR vector. **(A)** A chimeric gene sequence of a third-generation CAR. A third-generation CAR incorporates two different costimulatory molecules, typically CD28 and 4I-BB or OX40, expressed in tandem. The combinations in tandem costimulatory molecule expression can vary, for example, 4I-BB can be cloned to express upstream of fused CD28 and CD3ζ signaling domain or vice versa. **(B)** Chimeric third-generation CAR expression in T cells. **(C)** A magnified view of a typical third-generation CAR when expressed in T cells. **(D–F)** A third-generation two chain vector CAR. A third-generation chimeric gene sequence can be cloned to express two chains instead of one chain using a 2A cloning strategy. Basically, 2A can be used to separately express two tandemly cloned CARs: each CAR when expressed in T cells can possess an ectodomain, one costimulatory molecule, and an endodomain. The advantage of this strategy is that instead of fusing two costimulatory molecules together in a single chain, each costimulatory molecule can be cloned on separate chains. This cloning strategy can allow various modifications in two chain CARs, for example, one chain can be cloned to encode a signaling domain whereas another chain can be cloned to express signaling domains.

have scFv fused with costimulatory molecule and CD3ζ endodomain, whereas another chain may produce scFv fused with costimulatory molecule without CD3ζ endodomain (Fig. 2.4F) [28–32]. In addition, to enhance the potency of CARs novel transgenes have also been incorporated into the design of CARs such as cytokines *IL15*, cytokine receptor genes *IL15Rα* [33] as well as chemokine receptor genes. For example, the chemokine receptor gene *CCR4* has been incorporated to enhance trafficking of the CD30-CAR to target Hodgkin lymphoma [34]. Moreover, antiapoptotic genes *Bcl$_{XL}$* and *FLIP$_L$* have also been fused with the CAR sequences to avoid activation-induced cell death in second- and third-generation CARs (Balkhi MY and Junghans RP unpublished findings). Furthermore, to avoid on-target/off-tumor toxicity and cytokine storm syndrome, CARs have been modified with suicide genes such as herpes simplex virus-thymiding kinase *(HSV-TK)*. The cloning of caspase 9 *(iCasp9)* transgene safety switch with GD2-CAR has allowed depletion of disproportionally activated melanoma antigen-specific CAR-T cells in preclinical studies [35,36]. The inducible expression of iCasp9 depends on the administration of inhibitor drug AP1903. Taken together, these modifications in the basic CAR design have enhanced CAR potency. These will be further discussed in detail in Chapter 5.

CAR Ectodomain

The choice of antigen-binding ectodomain for CARs remain scFv. The variable heavy and variable light chain domains of scFvs are derived from two different gene segments linked by glycine-rich polypeptide linker (Fig. 2.1B). The linker provides flexibility and allows independent folding of variable light and heavy chains. The scFv-based CARs have demonstrated superior antigen affinity, effector functions, and cytokine secretion presumably due to scFv aggregation at the cell membrane [37]. ScFvs play a significant role in determining CARs' high or low antigen affinity,

on-target/off-tumor toxicity and overall antitumor responses. There have been educated attempts to express two scFvs targeting two different antigens. The two antibody scFv fragments are separated often by repeat glycine-serine linkers (glycin$_4$ serine)$_2$ or (glycin$_4$ serine)$_4$ then linked with a single hinge [5,38] (Fig. 2.5). Several bispecific CARs have been generated among which the human adenocarcinoma antigen CEA-TAG72 targeting CAR have demonstrated efficient antigen binding and killing of TAG72 expressing Jurkat and carcinoembryonic antigen (CEA) expressing rodent cell lines [39]. The idea behind dual specificity or bispecific CARs has been to increase the chance for better tumor-specific targeting and reducing the tumor escape mechanisms [39,40]. For example, CD19-CD20 bispecific CARs have demonstrated cytotoxicity against CD19$^+$ B-cell lymphoma as well as CD19$^-$ B-cell lymphoma through CD20 targeting [41]. However, whether the bispecific scFvs can produce synergistic or redundant effect on T-cell activity remains unclear. Moreover, it may not be unconceivable to assume that compared to monospecific CARs, the bispecific CARs could produce strong tonic signaling, and even with a small antigenic load, dual antigen targeting may produce strong persistent activation rendering bispecific CARs more prone to exhaustion. Furthermore, the production of bispecific CARs remains technically very challenging due to protein misfolding and solubility issues [42]. The clinical utility of bispecific CARs is further discussed in Chapter 5.

In addition to scFv or cytokine CARs, CARs composed of CD4 ectodomain fused to CD3ζ signaling domain have also been generated to target latent HIV1 infection reservoirs. The idea being that the extracellular domain of CD4 will allow recognizing gp120 of HIV envelope antigen. Both first- and second-generation CD4-targeting CARs have been generated [43–45]. The first-generation CD4 CAR expresses all four Ig-like domains of mature CD4 molecule as ectodomain.

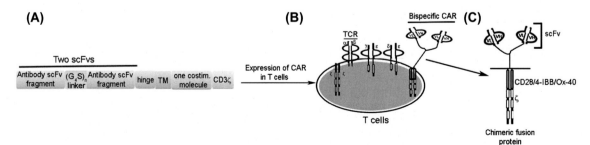

FIG. 2.5 A bispecific CAR. **(A–C)** The domain structures of a bispecific CAR. A bispecific CAR is cloned to express two antigen-binding scFvs separated by a glycine-rich linker sequence. The scFvs in a bispecific CAR can be encoded to recognize two different tumor-associated antigens.

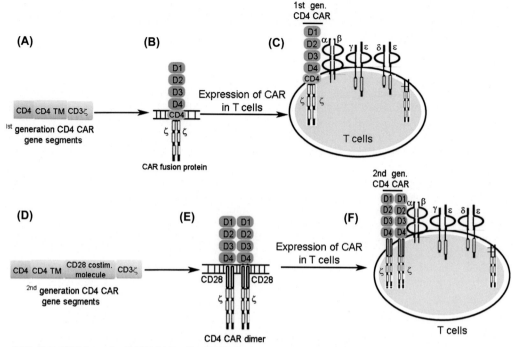

FIG. 2.6 CD4-based anti-HIV CARs. **(A–C)** The structure of a typical CD4 first-generation anti-HIV CAR. The CD4 CARs apart from anti-HIV CD4 molecule, which possess four-variable immunoglobulin-like domains, incorporates a CD4-derived transmembrane domain and a signaling domain, for example, CD3ζ. Anti-HIV CD4 CAR is capable of recognizing gp120 antigen on HIV1-infected cells. **(D–F)** The structure of a second-generation anti-HIV CAR that incorporates CD4 molecule fused to a costimulatory molecule typically CD28. The second-generation anti-HIV CD4 CARs usually dimerizes and is expressed on cell surface as a dimer.

The amino acid residues 372–395 of mature CD4 span the transmembrane domain, which is further fused with the CD3ζ signaling domain [43] (Fig. 2.6A–C). The second-generation CD4 CAR incorporates membrane tethered CD28 costimulatory molecule fused to CD3ζ signaling domain that causes dimerization of chimeric molecule [45] (Fig. 2.6D–F). It is worth noting that CD4 CARs are designed to be transduced through retroviral infections to modify CD8 CTL cells to achieve eradication of latent HIV1 infections through recognizing gp120 envelope protein. The advantage of CD4 CARs is that it can allow universal targeting of HIV1-infected CD4 T cells through antigen binding that is independent of HLA presentation. These CD4 CARs have demonstrated efficient cytokine production and cytolytic activity against HIV1-infected CD4 cells in ex vivo experiments [43]. However, they remain untested in humans and come with a distinct disadvantage as expression of CD4-CAR in CD8 T cells render these readily susceptible to HIV infection with virus binding and entry via CD4 ectodomain.

In addition to the scFv-based first-generation CARs, the CARs containing entire Fab fragment (Fig. 2.1A) including CH1 domains fused with CD3ζ or CD3ε signaling domains have also been created [5]. The CEA-specific Fab expressing first-generation CARs were tested against CEA expressing tumors and showed similar characteristics to that of CEA-scFvs [5]. Generally, scFv sequences are obtained from previously characterized antibody sequences and evaluated for affinity binding to tumor-associated or tumor-specific human antigens. However, most of the scFv sequences are derived from mouse strains, for example, the most famous CD19 scFv, which is generated from hybridoma FMC63 [46]. Even though the CARs produced these days are fully humanized still they remain at risk of producing antiidiotype mouse antibodies in the human host. There have been attempts to overcome this risk by using Camelid-derived antibodies. Camelid-produced antibodies possess single-variable domain heavy chain (VHH or nanobodies), a single CH1 domain but lack entirely the light chains. Camelid-derived antibodies are versatile antigen-binding molecules [47], and possess high stability and solubility. Due to their close homology with human VH antibody chain, these VHHs demonstrated extremely low immunogenicity offering an alternate choice to scFv in designing CARs [48]. In addition to scFvs, T-cell receptors have been modified to express specific cytokine genes such as IL13 cytokine [49]. The first-generation IL13 CAR was constructed by introducing mutated IL13 sequence IL13 (E13Y) with a chimeric hinge composed of human GM-CSFRα and immunoglobulin G4 (IgG4). The hinge was fused with transmembrane domain derived from human CD4 glycoprotein, which was further fused with cytoplasmic CD3ζ signaling domain (Fig. 2.7A−C). The idea to introduce mutant IL13 (E13Y) was intended to reduce binding to IL13Rα1/IL4Rα and increase specific targeting of IL13Rα2 expressing glioblastoma (GB) multiforme cancer [50]. An estimated 50% patients affected with GB express IL13Rα2, which is usually associated with poor

prognosis [51,52]. In an additional modification to the previously clinically tested IL13 CAR [50], costimulatory domain of CD137 (4-IBB) molecule was incorporated with mutated IgG4-Fc (IL13BBζ-CAR T) linker (Fig. 2.7D−F). The purpose to use mutated IgG4-Fc in IL13Rα2-targeting CAR has been to reduce off-target binding to Fc receptors. The IL13 CARs similar to scFv-based CARs have shown efficient cytokine production, proliferative capacity and persistence, and have shown remarkable success in early clinical trials [53−55]. Taken together, the utility of cytokine-based CARs may be limited to rare cancers due to lack of specific cytokine receptor targets in cancers. However, chemokine receptor targeting of tumors through chemokine CARs may provide a useful alternative.

Significance of Choosing Antibody Domains (CARbodies) for the CARs

Antibody domains provide CAR-modified T cells with power to hunt down tumors and viral infections.

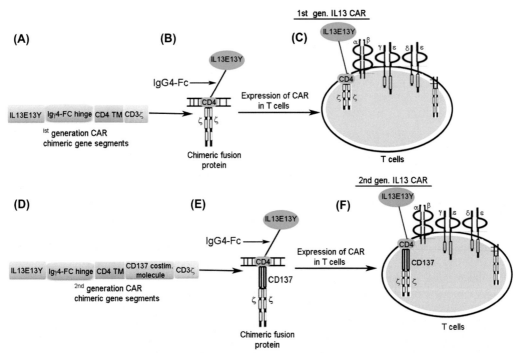

FIG. 2.7 Schematic representation of first- and second-generation anti-IL13 CAR designed to target IL13Rα2-positive glioblastoma (GB). **(A−C)** Design of first-generation IL13-CAR. The mutation IL13 (E13Y) was introduced to increase specific binding to IL13Rα2-positive glioblastoma and reduce binding to IL13Rα1/IL4Rα. The first-generation IL13-CAR does not possess costimulatory molecule, the ectodomain is linked to CD3ζ signaling domain through CD4 transmembrane domain. **(D−F)** Design of second-generation IL13-CAR. The second-generation IL13-CAR incorporates 4I-BB (CD137) or CD28 costimulatory molecule fused to CD3ζ signaling domain.

Therefore, selection of an antibody predominantly scFv for antigen targeting is pivotal for the therapeutic success of CARs. Choice of selecting antigen-specific antibody domain (hereafter CARbodies) for CARs is determined by several factors: (1) choice of an antigen; (2) affinity maturation of an antibody in vivo; (3) correct expression of three-dimensional structure of antibody domains on the surface of T cells; and (4) an in silico prediction that could help minimizing on-target/on-tumor and off-tumor toxicities. Antibodies raised against tumor neoantigens or cancer germline genes would have been ideal for CARs because such antibodies would recognize tumor-specific antigens without involving the risk of on-target/off-tumor toxicities often observed with CARs targeting tumor-associated self-antigens. However, choosing an antigen-specific antibody domain is often limited by the lack of expression of neoantigens or cancer germline genes on cancers except for rare immune reactive cancers such as melanoma or renal cell carcinoma and virally induced cancers that are known to express tumor-specific antigens [56,57]. Especially, the cancer germline genes such as members of the melanoma antigen *MAGE A, B* or *C* families and *LAGE* family genes expressed by melanoma [58] offer an excellent choice to generate CARbodies. Intense efforts are being devoted to whole-exome sequencing and RNA-Seq analysis on tumors to identify novel tumor antigens that potentially could be exploited to develop novel and better CARs for eliciting tumor-specific T-cell responses [59–62].

CARbodies are generally produced against tumor-associated antigens (TAAs). TAAs are also expressed by the normal tissues. Therefore, an antibody suboptimal avidity for tumor-associated antigens can increase the risk of on-target/off-tumor toxicities. In addition to protein antigens, CARbodies can also be raised against carbohydrates and glycolipids that could significantly increase the choice of antigenic targets for CARs [63]. Overall, for the therapeutic success, a CAR must express antibody domains with optimal avidity for tumor antigens and must present correctly the three-dimensional chimeric protein structure. Accordingly, CARs are intensively tested and validated for these properties in preclinical models.

Most antibody domains used in CAR design are IgG based and mouse derived. The tumor-associated antigen-specific antibodies especially scFvs for CARs are readily generated through immunization of mice. Historically, however, the first scFv antibody was cloned in pRSV2 expression vector containing the rearranged genes encoding scFv of heavy and light chains of SP6,

a monoclonal anti-2,4,6-trinitrophenyl (TNP) antibody. The anti-TNP scFv was successfully expressed on a CTL hybridoma line and successfully triggered hapten-specific target lysis and cytokine production [2]. Hwu, P. et al., were the first to construct the scFv-based CAR that targeted genuine cancer antigen, the folate-binding protein expressed in ovarian cancer. Moreover, the antifolate-binding CAR demonstrated tumor-specific cytotoxicity and effector cytokine production in vitro [3]. Since then scFv-based CARs have been routinely designed, constructed and validated for effector functions.

Even though the CARbodies have shown great success in eradicating lymphomas, they come with several caveats especially related to MHC-independent responses to tumor and viral antigens: (1) CARbody-mediated antigen recognition is MHC independent and may deprive T cells of help from professional antigen-presenting cells that potentially could deliver more potent antigenic responses; (2) CARbodies are specialized to respond to membrane-bound antigens, whereas soluble antigens and neoantigens that may be presented through MHC class I by the tumors essentially escape CAR recognition; (3) CARbodies are generally monoclonal antibodies that are designed to recognize a unique tumor antigen, which is one limitation with CARs, while tumors usually have high mutation rates, CARbodies in T cells essentially lack somatic hypermutation capacity to diversify CARbody antigen-binding domains [64]. Therefore, tumor and viral antigens may escape CAR recognition.

Choice of Hinges Supporting scFvs

In addition to antigen-binding domains, hinge plays a crucial role in CAR functions. The importance of hinge region was demonstrated in a study in which three scFv CARs were generated to target ErbB-2 receptor. Two ErbB-2-specific scFvs were fused to CD3ζ through a hinge while one was directly linked to CD3ζ without a hinge. Compared to hingeless ErbB-2 scFV, hinge containing scFvs exhibited antigen binding, lysed ERbB-2 expressing tumors, and excreted cytokines demonstrating the utility of hinge for CAR effector functions [65]. Hinges because of their importance for CAR functions have undergone several modifications as discussed below. Hinge is usually incorporated into CAR design to provide flexibility to the scFv antigen-binding domains and help avoiding steric hindrance [32,66]. Hinge is usually composed of CD8α chain or constant CH2–CH3 regions of IgG1, IgG4, or IgG3 [39]. It is worth noting that hinge requirement is most needed when CARs are linked to CD3ζ signaling domains. In contrast, CARs linked with ITAMs derived from FcεRI-γ chain does not need hinge. It has been reported that some cases including hinge may hinder CAR functions [67,68]. A direct comparison in effector functions was made between hingeless and hinge (derived from IgG1 CH2–CH3) containing CARs. CARs with CH2–CH3 hinge such as 5T4 and CD19 showed superior effector functions compared to CEA and neural cell adhesion molecule (NCAM) hingeless CARs that showed in comparison suboptimal activity [69]. When variable length hinges derived from IgG4-Fc were compared for effector activity in the receptor tyrosine kinase-like orphan receptor 1 (ROR1) specific third-generation CARs, a shorter length hinge showed superior killing of B-cell chronic lymphocyte leukemia cell lines ectopically expressing ROR1+ tumors compared to longer CH2–CH3 hinge [30]. These results demonstrate that utilizing an optimal hinge length can improve CAR-mediated tumor cytotoxicity.

Choice of CAR Transmembrane Domains

All CARs possess a transmembrane domain. The transmembrane domain is usually composed of CD4, CD8, CD3ζ domains or domains derived from costimulatory molecules. The requirement of transmembrane domain is essential for preserving the stability of CARs and for intracellular signaling. An optimal intracellular signaling strength is crucial for T-cell activation and cytokine production. The transmembrane domain composed of CD3ζ has been shown to lead optimal activation of CAR-T cells in direct comparison with MHC class I transmembrane domain [70,71]. Moreover, the Jurkat T cells modified with CEA-specific CARs and expressing CD3ζ transmembrane domain have shown optimal activation, antitumor functions, and cytokine production. The optimal activation of CAR-modified Jurkat T was attributed to the ability of CD3ζ transmembrane domain to induce heterodimerization of CAR molecules with the endogenous CD3ζ molecules of TCR-CD3 complex. A further proof of this effect was provided by experiments that showed an abrogation of activity when a mutated CD3ζ transmembrane was expressed [70]. Additional evidences about CD3ζ transmembrane domain inducing dimerization and optimal activation were provided by the Brentjens et al., who reported the homodimerization of CD19-CD3ζ CARs [72]. The importance of the choice of transmembrane domains was further demonstrated in a study that demonstrated first-generation CD19-CAR having a portion of CD3ζ expressed as transmembrane domain to be lacking viability and persistence in vivo than the second-generation CD19-CARs having

CD28 costimulatory molecule incorporated as a transmembrane domain [72,73]. In addition to CD3ζ, CD4 and CD8 domains have also been incorporated as transmembrane domains. The first-generation CARs incorporating CD4 or CD8 sequences expressed as transmembrane domains demonstrated no major differences in cytokine synthesis [74]. However, swapping CD4 transmembrane domain with CD28 in CD4 CARs designed to target HIV gp120 envelope protein demonstrated increased activation, cytolysis of infected cells, and enhanced cytokine production possibly through inducing homodimerization of chimeric molecules [45]. Therefore, apart from the structural value, the choice of transmembrane domain can also alter the functionality of CARs. Overall, expressing CD3ζ and CD28 molecules as transmembrane domains of CARs remains a popular choice.

Choice of CAR Endodomains and Costimulatory Molecules

To initiate strong intracellular signaling after TCR/MHC-antigen interaction, T cells depend on CD3 accessory molecules. The CD3ζ homodimer undergoes phosphorylation at conserved tyrosine residues within cytoplasmic domains of immunoreceptor tyrosine-based transactivation motifs (ITAMs) [75,76]. The phosphorylated tyrosine residues with CD3ζ chain couple with ZAP70. ZAP70 phosphorylates tyrosine residues in Lat and SLP76 to help recruit adapter proteins. Adaptor protein complex subsequently disperses and activates downstream signaling pathways to activate gene transcription program important for generating an optimal T-cell response. Therefore, CAR ectodomain after antigen recognition must be able to initiate intracellular signaling events strong enough to evoke tyrosine phosphorylation and gene transcription program for generating antitumor responses. The CD3ζ signaling molecule forms a natural choice. Not long after the first report of CD3ζ cloning and expression [77], the idea to test the feasibility of using CD3ζ as a signaling domain for CARs gained attention. The CD3ζ as choice of signaling domain for CARs forms an integral component of CAR T-cell technology today. The CD3ζ signaling domain has been incorporated into the design of commercially and clinically successful CARs [31,78–80]. Along with the CD3ζ, Fc receptor for IgE, the FcεRIγ, possesses ITAMs; however, it contains only one ITAM as opposed to three in CD3ζ chain but each contain paired YxxL/I motifs separated by six to eight variable amino acid residues [81,82]. Nevertheless, ITAMs of FcεRI and FcγRI like the CD3ζ recruits ZAP70 and other protein tyrosine kinases and couple the adaptors with downstream signaling molecules [83,84]. The FcεRI and FcγRI, therefore, offers an additional choice to be used as signaling domains for the CARs.

REFERENCES

[1] Gross G, Gorochov G, Waks T, Eshhar Z. Generation of effector T cells expressing chimeric T cell receptor with antibody type-specificity. Transplant Proc 1989;21: 127–30.

[2] Gross G, Waks T, Eshhar Z. Expression of immunoglobulin-T-cell receptor chimeric molecules as functional receptors with antibody-type specificity. Proc Natl Acad Sci USA 1989;86:10024–8.

[3] Hwu P, Shafer GE, Treisman J, Schindler DG, Gross G, Cowherd R, et al. Lysis of ovarian cancer cells by human lymphocytes redirected with a chimeric gene composed of an antibody variable region and the Fc receptor gamma chain. J Exp Med 1993;178:361–6.

[4] Hartmann J, Schussler-Lenz M, Bondanza A, Buchholz CJ. Clinical development of CAR T cells-challenges and opportunities in translating innovative treatment concepts. EMBO Mol Med 2017;9:1183–97.

[5] Nolan KF, Yun CO, Akamatsu Y, Murphy JC, Leung SO, Beecham EJ, et al. Bypassing immunization: optimized design of "designer T cells" against carcinoembryonic antigen (CEA)-expressing tumors, and lack of suppression by soluble CEA. Clin Cancer Res 1999;5:3928–41.

[6] Yun CO, Nolan KF, Beecham EJ, Reisfeld RA, Junghans RP. Targeting of T lymphocytes to melanoma cells through chimeric anti-GD3 immunoglobulin T-cell receptors. Neoplasia 2000;2:449–59.

[7] Beecham EJ, Ortiz-Pujols S, Junghans RP. Dynamics of tumor cell killing by human T lymphocytes armed with an anti-carcinoembryonic antigen chimeric immunoglobulin T-cell receptor. J Immunother 2000;23:332–43.

[8] Elliott BE, Carlow DA, Rodricks AM, Wade A. Perspectives on the role of MHC antigens in normal and malignant cell development. Adv Cancer Res 1989;53:181–245.

[9] D'Urso CM, Wang ZG, Cao Y, Tatake R, Zeff RA, Ferrone S. Lack of HLA class I antigen expression by cultured melanoma cells FO-1 due to a defect in B2m gene expression. J Clin Invest 1991;87:284–92.

[10] Restifo NP, Esquivel F, Kawakami Y, Yewdell JW, Mule JJ, Rosenberg SA, et al. Identification of human cancers deficient in antigen processing. J Exp Med 1993;177:265–72.

[11] Wolfram RM, Budinsky AC, Brodowicz T, Kubista M, Kostler WJ, Kichler-Lakomy C, et al. Defective antigen presentation resulting from impaired expression of costimulatory molecules in breast cancer. Int J Cancer 2000;88: 239–44.

[12] Seliger B, Harders C, Wollscheid U, Staege MS, Reske-Kunz AB, Huber C. Suppression of MHC class I antigens in oncogenic transformants: association with decreased recognition by cytotoxic T lymphocytes. Exp Hematol 1996;24:1275–9.

[13] Schwartz JC, Zhang X, Nathenson SG, Almo SC. Structural mechanisms of costimulation. Nat Immunol 2002;3: 427–34.

[14] Schwartz RH. T cell anergy. Annu Rev Immunol 2003;21: 305–34.

[15] Crespo J, Sun H, Welling TH, Tian Z, Zou W. T cell anergy, exhaustion, senescence, and stemness in the tumor microenvironment. Curr Opin Immunol 2013;25: 214–21.

[16] Driessens G, Kline J, Gajewski TF. Costimulatory and coinhibitory receptors in anti-tumor immunity. Immunol Rev 2009;229:126–44.

[17] Kershaw MH, Teng MW, Smyth MJ, Darcy PK. Supernatural T cells: genetic modification of T cells for cancer therapy. Nat Rev Immunol 2005;5:928–40.

[18] Scholler J, Brady TL, Binder-Scholl G, Hwang WT, Plesa G, Hege KM, et al. Decade-long safety and function of retroviral-modified chimeric antigen receptor T cells. Sci Transl Med 2012;4:132ra53.

[19] Wang X, Naranjo A, Brown CE, Bautista C, Wong CW, Chang WC, et al. Phenotypic and functional attributes of lentivirus-modified CD19-specific human CD8$^+$ central memory T cells manufactured at clinical scale. J Immunother 2012;35:689–701.

[20] Kebriaei P, Huls H, Jena B, Munsell M, Jackson R, Lee DA, et al. Infusing CD19-directed T cells to augment disease control in patients undergoing autologous hematopoietic stem-cell transplantation for advanced B-lymphoid malignancies. Hum Gene Ther 2012;23:444–50.

[21] Singh H, Manuri PR, Olivares S, Dara N, Dawson MJ, Huls H, et al. Redirecting specificity of T-cell populations for CD19 using the Sleeping Beauty system. Cancer Res 2008;68:2961–71.

[22] June CH, Blazar BR, Riley JL. Engineering lymphocyte subsets: tools, trials and tribulations. Nat Rev Immunol 2009;9:704–16.

[23] aiti SN, Huls H, Singh H, Dawson M, Figliola M, Olivares S, et al. Sleeping beauty system to redirect T-cell specificity for human applications. J Immunother 2013;36:112–23.

[24] Huls MH, Figliola MJ, Dawson MJ, Olivares S, Kebriaei P, Shpall EJ, et al. Clinical application of Sleeping Beauty and artificial antigen presenting cells to genetically modify T cells from peripheral and umbilical cord blood. J Vis Exp 2013:e50070.

[25] Singh H, Figliola MJ, Dawson MJ, Olivares S, Zhang L, Yang G, et al. Manufacture of clinical-grade CD19-specific T cells stably expressing chimeric antigen receptor using Sleeping Beauty system and artificial antigen presenting cells. PLoS One 2013;8:e64138.

[26] Jena B, Dotti G, Cooper LJ. Redirecting T-cell specificity by introducing a tumor-specific chimeric antigen receptor. Blood 2010;116:1035–44.

[27] Kershaw MH, Westwood JA, Parker LL, Wang G, Eshhar Z, Mavroukakis SA, et al. A phase I study on adoptive immunotherapy using gene-modified T cells for ovarian cancer. Clin Cancer Res 2006;12:6106–15.

[28] Ma Q, Gonzalo-Daganzo RM, Junghans RP. Genetically engineered T cells as adoptive immunotherapy of cancer. Cancer Chemother Biol Response Modif 2002; 20:315−41.

[29] Dotti G, Gottschalk S, Savoldo B, Brenner MK. Design and development of therapies using chimeric antigen receptor-expressing T cells. Immunol Rev 2014;257: 107−26.

[30] Hudecek M, Lupo-Stanghellini MT, Kosasih PL, Sommermeyer D, Jensen MC, Rader C, et al. Receptor affinity and extracellular domain modifications affect tumor recognition by ROR1-specific chimeric antigen receptor T cells. Clin Cancer Res 2013;19:3153−64.

[31] Brentjens RJ, Davila ML, Riviere I, Park J, Wang X, Cowell LG, et al. CD19-targeted T cells rapidly induce molecular remissions in adults with chemotherapy-refractory acute lymphoblastic leukemia. Sci Transl Med 2013;5:177ra38.

[32] Sadelain M, Brentjens R, Riviere I. The basic principles of chimeric antigen receptor design. Cancer Discov 2013;3: 388−98.

[33] Hurton LV, Singh H, Najjar AM, Switzer KC, Mi T, Maiti S, et al. Tethered IL-15 augments antitumor activity and promotes a stem-cell memory subset in tumor-specific T cells. Proc Natl Acad Sci USA 2016;113:E7788−97.

[34] Di Stasi A, De Angelis B, Rooney CM, Zhang L, Mahendravada A, Foster AE, et al. T lymphocytes coexpressing CCR4 and a chimeric antigen receptor targeting CD30 have improved homing and antitumor activity in a Hodgkin tumor model. Blood 2009;113:6392−402.

[35] Hoyos V, Savoldo B, Quintarelli C, Mahendravada A, Zhang M, Vera J, et al. Engineering CD19-specific T lymphocytes with interleukin-15 and a suicide gene to enhance their anti-lymphoma/leukemia effects and safety. Leukemia 2010;24:1160−70.

[36] Gargett T, Brown MP. The inducible caspase-9 suicide gene system as a "safety switch" to limit on-target, off-tumor toxicities of chimeric antigen receptor T cells. Front Pharmacol 2014;5:235.

[37] Chmielewski M, Hombach A, Heuser C, Adams GP, Abken H. T cell activation by antibody-like immunoreceptors: increase in affinity of the single-chain fragment domain above threshold does not increase T cell activation against antigen-positive target cells but decreases selectivity. J Immunol 2004;173:7647−53.

[38] Martyniszyn A, Krahl AC, Andre MC, Hombach AA, Abken H. CD20-CD19 bispecific CAR T cells for the treatment of B-cell malignancies. Hum Gene Ther 2017;28: 1147−57.

[39] Patel SD, Moskalenko M, Tian T, Smith D, McGuinness R, Chen L, et al. T-cell killing of heterogenous tumor or viral targets with bispecific chimeric immune receptors. Cancer Gene Ther 2000;7:1127−34.

[40] Grada Z, Hegde M, Byrd T, Shaffer DR, Ghazi A, Brawley VS, et al. TanCAR: a novel bispecific chimeric antigen receptor for cancer immunotherapy. Mol Ther Nucleic Acids 2013;2:e105.

[41] Zah E, Lin MY, Silva-Benedict A, Jensen MC, Chen YY. T cells expressing CD19/CD20 bispecific chimeric antigen receptors prevent antigen escape by malignant B cells. Cancer Immunol Res 2016;4:498−508.

[42] Kuhlman B, Baker D. Exploring folding free energy landscapes using computational protein design. Curr Opin Struct Biol 2004;14:89−95.

[43] Roberts MR, Qin L, Zhang D, Smith DH, Tran AC, Dull TJ, et al. Targeting of human immunodeficiency virus-infected cells by CD8+ T lymphocytes armed with universal T-cell receptors. Blood 1994;84:2878−89.

[44] Yang OO, Tran AC, Kalams SA, Johnson RP, Roberts MR, Walker BD. Lysis of HIV-1-infected cells and inhibition of viral replication by universal receptor T cells. Proc Natl Acad Sci USA 1997;94:11478−83.

[45] Sahu GK, Sango K, Selliah N, Ma Q, Skowron G, Junghans RP. Anti-HIV designer T cells progressively eradicate a latently infected cell line by sequentially inducing HIV reactivation then killing the newly gp120-positive cells. Virology 2013;446:268−75.

[46] Nicholson IC, Lenton KA, Little DJ, Decorso T, Lee FT, Scott AM, et al. Construction and characterisation of a functional CD19 specific single chain Fv fragment for immunotherapy of B lineage leukaemia and lymphoma. Mol Immunol 1997;34:1157−65.

[47] Hamers-Casterman C, Atarhouch T, Muyldermans S, Robinson G, Hamers C, Songa EB, et al. Naturally occurring antibodies devoid of light chains. Nature 1993;363: 446−8.

[48] Harmsen MM, De Haard HJ. Properties, production, and applications of camelid single-domain antibody fragments. Appl Microbiol Biotechnol 2007;77:13−22.

[49] Kahlon KS, Brown C, Cooper LJ, Raubitschek A, Forman SJ, Jensen MC. Specific recognition and killing of glioblastoma multiforme by interleukin 13-zetakine redirected cytolytic T cells. Cancer Res 2004;64:9160−6.

[50] Brown CE, Badie B, Barish ME, Weng L, Ostberg JR, Chang WC, et al. Bioactivity and safety of IL13Ralpha2-redirected chimeric antigen receptor CD8+ T cells in patients with recurrent glioblastoma. Clin Cancer Res 2015;21:4062−72.

[51] Brown CE, Starr R, Aguilar B, Shami AF, Martinez C, D'Apuzzo M, et al. Stem-like tumor-initiating cells isolated from IL13Ralpha2 expressing gliomas are targeted and killed by IL13-zetakine-redirected T Cells. Clin Cancer Res 2012;18:2199−209.

[52] Debinski W, Gibo DM, Hulet SW, Connor JR, Gillespie GY. Receptor for interleukin 13 is a marker and therapeutic target for human high-grade gliomas. Clin Cancer Res 1999;5:985−90.

[53] Sengupta S, Thaci B, Crawford AC, Sampath P. Interleukin-13 receptor alpha 2-targeted glioblastoma immunotherapy. Biomed Res Int 2014;2014:952128.

[54] Thaci B, Brown CE, Binello E, Werbaneth K, Sampath P, Sengupta S. Significance of interleukin-13 receptor alpha 2-targeted glioblastoma therapy. Neuro Oncol 2014;16: 1304−12.

[55] Brown CE, Alizadeh D, Starr R, Weng L, Wagner JR, Naranjo A, et al. Regression of glioblastoma after chimeric antigen receptor T-cell therapy. N Engl J Med 2016;375:2561–9.

[56] Rosenberg SA. Progress in human tumour immunology and immunotherapy. Nature 2001;411:380–4.

[57] Heslop HE, Ng CY, Li C, Smith CA, Loftin SK, Krance RA, et al. Long-term restoration of immunity against Epstein-Barr virus infection by adoptive transfer of gene-modified virus-specific T lymphocytes. Nat Med 1996;2:551–5.

[58] van der Bruggen P, Traversari C, Chomez P, Lurquin C, De Plaen E, Van den Eynde B, et al. A gene encoding an antigen recognized by cytolytic T lymphocytes on a human melanoma. Science 1991;254:1643–7.

[59] Robbins PF, Lu YC, El-Gamil M, Li YF, Gross C, Gartner J, et al. Mining exomic sequencing data to identify mutated antigens recognized by adoptively transferred tumor-reactive T cells. Nat Med 2013;19:747–52.

[60] Lu YC, Yao X, Crystal JS, Li YF, El-Gamil M, Gross C, et al. Efficient identification of mutated cancer antigens recognized by T cells associated with durable tumor regressions. Clin Cancer Res 2014;20:3401–10.

[61] Coulie PG, Van den Eynde BJ, van der Bruggen P, Boon T. Tumour antigens recognized by T lymphocytes: at the core of cancer immunotherapy. Nat Rev Cancer 2014; 14:135–46.

[62] Stevanovic S, Pasetto A, Helman SR, Gartner JJ, Prickett TD, Howie B, et al. Landscape of immunogenic tumor antigens in successful immunotherapy of virally induced epithelial cancer. Science 2017;356:200–5.

[63] Mezzanzanica D, Canevari S, Mazzoni A, Figini M, Colnaghi MI, Waks T, et al. Transfer of chimeric receptor gene made of variable regions of tumor-specific antibody confers anticarbohydrate specificity on T cells. Cancer Gene Ther 1998;5:401–7.

[64] Wu X, Feng J, Komori A, Kim EC, Zan H, Casali P. Immunoglobulin somatic hypermutation: double-strand DNA breaks, AID and error-prone DNA repair. J Clin Immunol 2003;23:235–46.

[65] Moritz D, Groner B. A spacer region between the single chain antibody- and the CD3 zeta-chain domain of chimeric T cell receptor components is required for efficient ligand binding and signaling activity. Gene Ther 1995;2:539–46.

[66] Sadelain M, Riviere I, Brentjens R. Targeting tumours with genetically enhanced T lymphocytes. Nat Rev Cancer 2003;3:35–45.

[67] Hombach A, Heuser C, Gerken M, Fischer B, Lewalter K, Diehl V, et al. T cell activation by recombinant FcepsilonRI gamma-chain immune receptors: an extracellular spacer domain impairs antigen-dependent T cell activation but not antigen recognition. Gene Ther 2000;7:1067–75.

[68] Uherek C, Groner B, Wels W. Chimeric antigen receptors for the retargeting of cytotoxic effector cells. J Hematother Stem Cell Res 2001;10:523–34.

[69] Guest RD, Hawkins RE, Kirillova N, Cheadle EJ, Arnold J, O'Neill A, et al. The role of extracellular spacer regions in the optimal design of chimeric immune receptors: evaluation of four different scFvs and antigens. J Immunother 2005;28:203–11.

[70] Bridgeman JS, Hawkins RE, Bagley S, Blaylock M, Holland M, Gilham DE. The optimal antigen response of chimeric antigen receptors harboring the CD3zeta transmembrane domain is dependent upon incorporation of the receptor into the endogenous TCR/CD3 complex. J Immunol 2010;184:6938–49.

[71] Gilham DE, O'Neil A, Hughes C, Guest RD, Kirillova N, Lehane M, et al. Primary polyclonal human T lymphocytes targeted to carcino-embryonic antigens and neural cell adhesion molecule tumor antigens by CD3zeta-based chimeric immune receptors. J Immunother 2002; 25:139–51.

[72] Brentjens RJ, Latouche JB, Santos E, Marti F, Gong MC, Lyddane C, et al. Eradication of systemic B-cell tumors by genetically targeted human T lymphocytes co-stimulated by CD80 and interleukin-15. Nat Med 2003; 9:279–86.

[73] Savoldo B, Ramos CA, Liu E, Mims MP, Keating MJ, Carrum G, et al. CD28 costimulation improves expansion and persistence of chimeric antigen receptor-modified T cells in lymphoma patients. J Clin Investig 2011;121: 1822–6.

[74] Fitzer-Attas CJ, Schindler DG, Waks T, Eshhar Z. Harnessing Syk family tyrosine kinases as signaling domains for chimeric single chain of the variable domain receptors: optimal design for T cell activation. J Immunol 1998; 160:145–54.

[75] Davis MM. A new trigger for T cells. Cell 2002;110: 285–7.

[76] Zoller KE, MacNeil IA, Brugge JS. Protein tyrosine kinases Syk and ZAP-70 display distinct requirements for Src family kinases in immune response receptor signal transduction. J Immunol 1997;158:1650–9.

[77] Weissman AM, Baniyash M, Hou D, Samelson LE, Burgess WH, Klausner RD. Molecular cloning of the zeta chain of the T cell antigen receptor. Science 1988; 239:1018–21.

[78] Lee DW, Kochenderfer JN, Stetler-Stevenson M, Cui YK, Delbrook C, Feldman SA, et al. T cells expressing CD19 chimeric antigen receptors for acute lymphoblastic leukaemia in children and young adults: a phase 1 dose-escalation trial. Lancet 2015;385:517–28.

[79] Maude SL, Frey N, Shaw PA, Aplenc R, Barrett DM, Bunin NJ, et al. Chimeric antigen receptor T cells for sustained remissions in leukemia. N Engl J Med 2014;371: 1507–17.

[80] Sheridan C. First approval in sight for Novartis' CAR-T therapy after panel vote. Nat Biotechnol 2017;35: 691–3.

[81] Haynes NM, Snook MB, Trapani JA, Cerruti L, Jane SM, Smyth MJ, et al. Redirecting mouse CTL against colon carcinoma: superior signaling efficacy of single-chain variable domain chimeras containing TCR-zeta vs Fc epsilon RI-gamma. J Immunol 2001;166:182–7.

[82] Underhill DM, Goodridge HS. The many faces of ITAMs. Trends Immunol 2007;28:66−73.

[83] Indik ZK, Park JG, Hunter S, Schreiber AD. The molecular dissection of Fc gamma receptor mediated phagocytosis. Blood 1995;86:4389−99.

[84] Park JG, Schreiber AD. Determinants of the phagocytic signal mediated by the type IIIA Fc gamma receptor, Fc gamma RIIIA: sequence requirements and interaction with protein-tyrosine kinases. Proc Natl Acad Sci USA 1995;92:7381−5.

scFv Cloning, Vectors, and CAR-T Production in Laboratory for Preclinical Applications

ADVANTAGES OF USING SCFV OVER FULL-LENGTH MONOCLONAL ANTIBODY IN CAR THERAPY

The use of single-chain variable fragment (scFv) of an antibody for chimeric antigen receptors (CARs) comes with several advantages that a full-length monoclonal antibody cannot provide. Typically, an antibody is composed of four polypeptide chains, two light chains (length of a light chain is about $\sim$220 amino acids), and two heavy chains (length of a heavy chain is about $\sim$420 amino acids). These chains fold into distinct domains (Fig. 3.1A). The variable light and heavy chain interact through a disulphide bond forming an N-terminal antigen-binding domain. The variable light and heavy chain domains contain hypervariable (HV) and framework (FR) regions. There may be up to three HV regions whose amino acid sequences vary between antigen specific antibodies. The three hypervariable (HV) loops are supported by up to four framework (FR) regions whose amino acid sequences remain often stable. The papain enzyme digestion of all antibodies (except IgM and IgE) yield Fab fragments. The Fab fragments apart from variable domains contain the first constant heavy and light chain domains (Fig. 3.1A,B). The antibody heavy chain contains three to four (four in IgE and IgM antibodies) constant (C) domains. The C-terminal heavy chain constant domain form Fc region of antibodies that interacts with Fc receptors present on immune cells including natural killer cells, monocytes, macrophages, and dendritic cells [1]. Typically, T cells do not express Fc receptors. The full-length intact antibodies especially IgG isotype antibodies, therefore, retains the ability to bind to the Fc receptors as well as to fix complement proteins. It is not unconceivable that a full length antibody directed against tumors may bind to nontumor cells as well as can fix complement proteins through their heavy chain constant domains reducing the overall target specificity and tumor localization. Harwood et al. directly compared the tumor and normal tissue localization/distribution of an anti-CEA antibody F(ab)′2 fragment (Fig. 3.1C) versus intact antibody in mice. Their results demonstrated that compared to intact antibody, F(ab)′2 fragment showed superior tumor localization and cleared much faster from the normal tissue spaces [2]. Therefore, these properties can be useful when antibodies are planned to be used in therapeutic and clinical diagnostic applications such as radioimaging. A study by Wahl RL et al. demonstrated that the anti-CEA antibody F(ab)′2 fragment performed better than Fab fragment and an intact antibody when used for radioimaging of human colon carcinoma xenograft, indicating that F(ab)′2 fragment offers superior advantage in imaging and potentially in therapeutic applications [3]. The recombinant DNA technology seems the most feasible way to generate Fab or Fv domains (Fig. 3.1D) of an antibody for therapeutic applications. However, it was observed that Fv fragments undergo reassociation soon after they get expressed in *Escherichia coli*. Therefore, to avoid the problem with reassociation of Fv fragment of an antibody, Bird RE et al. constructed the first scFv of an anti-BGH IgG antibody. The scFv consisted of a single polypeptide chain synthesized from V_L and V_H sequences. The carboxyl terminus of V_L was linked with the amino terminus of V_H through a peptide linker [3]. However, the linker can also be synthesized to link amino terminus of V_L with the carboxy terminus of V_H (Fig. 3.1E). Including a linker in the Fv fragment avoided the reassociation when expressed in *E. coli*. The V_L and V_H domains linked through a peptide linker associate through covalent binding after folding in *E. coli*. The scFvs have demonstrated antigen affinities comparable with monoclonal antibodies. Moreover, scFvs come with an added advantage of their small sizes, antigen-specific target localization, reduced Fc-receptor associated nonspecific binding, and faster serum clearance.

Basics of Chimeric Antigen Receptor (CAR) Immunotherapy. https://doi.org/10.1016/B978-0-12-819573-4.00003-X

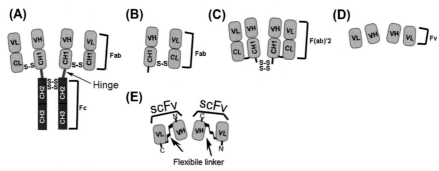

FIG. 3.1 Antibody domain structures. **(A)** Full-length antibody. **(B–C)** Fab and F(ab')2 fragment of antibody. **(D)** Variable heavy and light chain fragments (Fv). **(E)** Structure of single-chain variable fragment (scFv) used in the construction of CARs. ScFvs are basically variable heavy and light chain fragments connected through artificial linker.

CHOICES OF TUMOR ANTIGENS, THE MOLECULAR BIOLOGY TECHNIQUES USED TO GENERATE AND TEST TUMOR ANTIGEN-SPECIFIC SCFVS

Extensive in vivo data exist, as discussed previously in section Advantages of Using scFv Over Full-Length Monoclonal Antibody in CAR Therapy, that have demonstrated therapeutic benefits of utilizing scFvs over full-length antibodies. The next step toward producing CARs for clinical use is the construction of CAR chimeric gene sequences that includes apart from the *scFv*, the DNA sequences of a linker, a hinge, costimulatory molecule(s), and a signaling domain. However, the most critical and cumbersome component in CAR design is obtaining the DNA sequences for *scFv* cloning, and the functional characterization of scFvs. The construction of scFv involves the same steps as producing an antigen-specific antibody that begins with the best "choice of tumor antigen selection." The choice of tumor antigen for scFv generation is one of the most important steps in CAR therapy applications that eventually determines the clinical and commercial success of CARs. The intention for "commercial success" plays prominent role in guiding the choice of tumor antigens for scFv generation. Large biopharma companies have been investing billions of dollars in the CAR therapeutics. Moreover, some of these biopharma companies have bought smaller biotech companies or have been investing in sponsored research with the intention of commercializing the product. Therefore, commercial applicability guides in a big way the pharma decisions toward CAR generation and the choice of cancer targeting. For example, Biopharma companies that are investing in CAR therapeutics are mostly based in the United States, Europe, and Japan,

TABLE 3.1
Tumor Antigens Used for scFv Generation and Statistics About the Cancer Antigen-Associated Deaths.

Antigen	Tumor Antigen Prevalence	Antigen Tumor deaths/Year
Her2/neu	30% breast cancer	90,000–100,000
CEA	40% gastrointestinal	200,000–400,000
Mucin-1	60% pancreatic cancer	120,000
Mesothelin	100% pancreatic cancer	120,000
CD19	90% NHL	15,000
CD22	90% pediatric-ALL	1,400
CD22	90% NHL	15,000
LeY	70% lung cancer	100,000
MUC16	100% ovarian cancer	14,000

and as data demonstrate they have shown interest to target cancers that are more prevalent in the population, refractory to available treatments, and likely to cause significant cancer-related deaths such as breast cancer, pancreatic cancer [4–8], lymphoma [9,10], ovarian cancer [11], and lung cancer [12]. Table 3.1 provides the statistics about the cancers targeted with the CARs, choice of tumor antigens for scFv generation, and antigen-associated deaths (https://seer.cancer.gov/statistics/reports.html). The statistics about antigen specific deaths provided in Table 3.1 guide Biopharma and individual lab's pursuit for CAR-targeting of cancer.

CAR therapy is not limited by the antigenic targets but by the choice of tumor antigens. A tumor antigen that generates potent antitumor responses with minimal on-tumor/off-target toxicities makes for a best choice. As discussed in Chapter 1, Section 1.2.5, the tumor-associated self-antigens (TAA) have been the choice for CAR targeting and, as demonstrated in Table 3.1, most tumor antigens utilized for scFv generation are TAAs. Assuming a best choice of tumor antigen for CAR targeting has been made, the next step in CAR construction is the scFv generation that involves preparation and presentation of tumor antigens to the host (e.g., mice) in a form that generates powerful and antigen-specific antibody-mediated (humoral) immune responses.

scFv Generation Using Hybridoma

In the following sections, we will discuss how antigen-specific scFvs are generated and tested, which is the most crucial and cumbersome part of CAR production. Apart from the individual labs, several companies such as Creative Biolabs http://www.creative-biolabs.com/Chimeric-Antigen-Receptors-CARs.html offers services for custom scFv generation. Overall, scFv generation and validation can be achieved through (1) mice immunization and hybridoma generation, and (2) phage display techniques. Once a tumor antigen of choice, for example, carcinoembryonic antigen (CEA) or CD19 is made for CAR targeting of adenocarcinoma or B cell malignancies, the following procedure may be followed:

1. Immunization of mice. Selection of a mouse strain for immunization is crucial. For the preclinical studies, the choice of mice strain would not impose any problems. However, for generating scFv to be used in clinical studies in humans, a mouse-derived antibody might impose several problems. For example, mouse derived antibodies may show reduced potency due to cross-species reactivity and they may also pose additional risk of immunogenicity in the host. Therefore, so-called humanized mice are being increasingly used to generate fully humanized scFv for CARs. Two strategies are being used to produce fully humanized antibodies: (a) transgenic mice are engineered to carry human immunoglobulin (Ig) heavy and light chain gene segments in their germline, and endogenous *IgH* and *Igκ* locuses are disrupted rendering these mice incapable of producing mouse antibodies. The human *Ig* transgene in mouse germline reportedly undergo the processes of class switch recombination, V-D-J recombination and affinity maturation [13–15]. Affinity maturation represents one of the key features of this technology. Affinity maturation of an antibody refers to the process by which an antibody with highest affinity for an antigen is selected among the clone of antigen-specific antibodies generated in vivo. (b) A second strategy which is still evolving can also be applied to generate humanized antibodies. This strategy utilizes immunocompromised NSG mouse, NOD.Cg-*Prkdc^{scid}Il2rg^{tm1Wjl}*/SzJ (developed by Jackson laboratories, Bar Harbor, Strain id 005557). The NSG mice allows engraftment of human $CD34^+$ multipotent progenitors. That has shown to reconstitute in NSG mice a fully functional human immune system capable of generating T- and B-cell-mediated adaptive immune responses. Such mice generate tumor antigen-specific antibody responses when implanted with human cancer cells [16]. However, the hu-NSG mice are reported to have limited capacity to undergo class switch recombination and can only generate limited amount of human IgG. Nevertheless, if such deficiencies can be overcome, the hu-NSG mice offers an exciting opportunity to develop patient derived tumor antigen-specific hybridomas.

2. After immunization of humanized mice, spleens are harvested to isolate plasma B cells. It is to be noted, multiple cycles of immunizations protocols may be applied to induce affinity maturation for the production of high affinity antibodies.

3. Plasma cells are fused with myeloma cells to produce a hybridoma, which is screened for high affinity antibody production. At this stage, the antibody produced is full monoclonal antibody containing IgH and L chains.

4. The RNA is extracted from the hybridoma typically using 1×10^7 cells. This is followed by cDNA synthesis using reverse transcription method. cDNA is used as a template for PCR-mediated amplification of V_H and V_L gene segments using variable light and heavy chain frame work region specific primers [17] (Fig. 3.2A).

5. Subsequently, glycine-rich $(Gly_4Ser)_3$ linker sequences are inserted between the V_H and V_L genes sequences to construct scFv. At this stage, scFv sequence may be assembled in a phage display vector for further characterizations (shown in Fig. 3.2B).

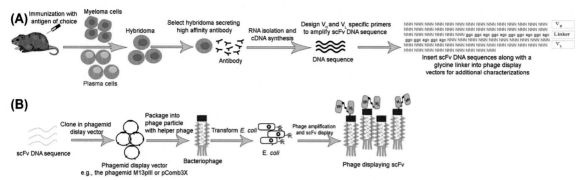

FIG. 3.2 Methods commonly used for generation and characterization of antigen-specific scFvs. **(A)** Shows immunization method utilized to produce antigen-specific hybridoma. Hybridoma are screened to identify high affinity antibody-producing clones. Multiple cycles of immunizations may be applied to induce antibody affinity maturation. ScFvs are derived from hybridoma clone by applying primers and gene amplifications. **(B)** Phage display technique summarizing steps involved in producing scFv libraries, their characterization such as scFv antigen-binding specificities, and elucidation of scFv three-dimensional structures.

scFv Screening Through Phage Display Technology

The phage display technology allows efficient screening and construction of high affinity scFv libraries. To generate a phage display library, the predetermined high affinity tumor antigen-specific scFv sequences are assembled. The scFv DNA sequence are inserted into a phage display vector, for example, the phagemid pComb3X, M13pIII. The phegemid may require separately helper phagemid, for example, M13KO7 for encoding a full bacteriophage [18]. The scFv genes are fused with the phage coat protein that allows scFv displaying in fusion with the phage coat protein. Once all the necessary phagemid plasmids are ready, following experimental approach is followed:

1. *E. coli* bacterial strains are transformed with the recombinant phagemid population to produce phage scFv library.
2. The scFv phage display library are screened with the specific antigens to identify and isolate target-specific antibody. Antigens are usually immobilized on ELISA plates.
3. The scFvs with optimized antibody affinity are sequenced to determine amino acid sequence and further characterizations follows with other parameters. Once the scFvs are fully characterized and essential parameters determined, these parameters can help choosing the scFv for CAR therapy. One more advantage of the phage display technology is that it allows production of fully human tumor antigen-specific scFvs. The sequencing of optimized

scFv may also help guiding the expression of fusion antibodies with epitope tagging such as poly-histidine or hemagglutinin tag for efficient purification [19]. A summary of procedure of antibody phage display is depicted in Fig. 3.2B.

Generating Chimeric Gene Sequences for Cloning Into Retroviral Vectors

Once all the functional parameters of scFv such as high affinity binding to the antigen and stable scFv-antigen interactions have been determined, the next step in the CAR construction is obtaining the DNA sequence of fully characterized scFv and the sequences of other CAR components that includes a linker, a hinge, transmembrane domain, costimulatory molecule, and a signaling domain (Fig. 3.3A). All these sequences are assembled and cloned into retroviral vectors, for example, pRSV2 vectors (Fig. 3.3B). The chimeric DNA sequences will be translated into amino acids (Fig. 3.3C), and a fully functional CAR fusion protein in virally transduced primary T cells will be expressed on its surface (Fig. 3.3D). The amino acid sequences of hinge and transmembrane domain (e.g., CD8α), costimulatory molecules (e.g., CD28), and signaling domains (e.g., CD3ζ) are available in various databases such as UniProt (https://www.uniprot.org/).

The other CAR chimeric gene sequences such as CD8α-hinge, CD8α-transmembrane domain, CD28 costimulatory domain, and CD3ζ signaling domain can be amplified from T cells using specific primers or can be custom synthesized. Taken together, all CAR chimeric gene sequences are assembled and cloned

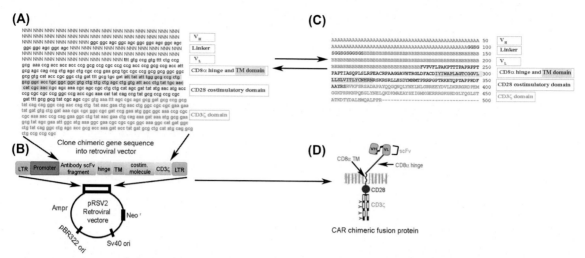

FIG. 3.3 DNA sequence of a typical CAR chimeric gene. **(A-B)** An assembled gene sequences of various components of CARs, the scFv (V_H, linker and V_L), CD8α-Hinge, CD8α-Transmembrane domain, CD28 costimulatory domain, and CD3ζ signaling domain used for cloning into expression vectors. Obtaining the antigen-specific scFv gene sequences (NNNNN ...) is the most important and tedious step in producing CARs. Once scFv sequences are confirmed, for example, through gene-sequencing techniques, the gene sequences of other components such as glycine-rich linker, transmembrane domains, costimulatory molecules, and intracellular signaling domains can be obtained from publicly available databases. These all are combined and cloned into expression vectors most commonly retroviral vectors **(B)**. **(C)** Protein sequence of a typical CAR once translated from cloned DNA sequences inside T cells (AAAA .... and BBBB .... represent unknown amino acid sequences of scFv whereas amino acid sequences of glycine-rich linker, CD8α hinge, transmembrane domains, CD28 costimulatory, and CD3ζ signaling domains are translated from the publicly available databases, for example, Uniprot. **(D)** CAR fusion protein structure after chimeric gene sequences cloned into retroviral vectors get translated inside the cells, often T cells.

into retroviral vectors (transfer plasmids), following which the retroviral vectors are transfected into packaging cell lines (vector-producing cell lines, e.g., PG13). The vector-producing cell lines will produce a pseudotyped virus with tropism for mammalian cells. The viral supernatants are collected and stored or used to infect primary human or mouse T cells. Following which, T cells will express CAR. The CAR-T cells can be subsequently tested for cancer target killings using cancer lines expressing CAR-specific tumor antigens or HLA-matched primary cancer cells. The scheme of the entire procedure is described (Fig. 3.4).

Retroviral Vectors Used for Cloning CAR Chimeric Genes

As we learned in above sections, the scFv chimeric gene sequences are assembled and inserted into retroviral vectors. These retroviral vectors are transfected into vector producer cell lines [e.g., PG13 or Phoenix or 293 [20,21]] for packaging chimeric genes into a replication-deficient virus. Once the virus is collected, these are utilized to infect primary human or mouse T

cells to produce CAR fusion protein for preclinical and clinical applications (Fig. 3.4). Therefore, the choice of vectors plays a vital role in CAR technology and eventual regulatory approvals for conducting clinical trials in humans. Today, most vectors used in CAR therapy are retroviral based. The potential application of retroviral-mediated gene transfer in humans had previously been successfully achieved in patients presented with inherited potentially lethal disorders [22–24]. Therefore, the potential application of retroviral-mediated gene transfer in CAR therapy for humans was realized very early. The choice of vectors-retroviral, lentiviral, or nonviral vectors- for cloning chimeric gene sequences and expression in producer cells, and finally T cell receptor modification for therapeutic applications forms an essential component of CAR T-cell technology. The choice of CAR vectors is therefore a major safety concern and assumes greater importance when the CARs are used for clinical trials and are in the pipeline for receiving FDA approvals. FDA guidelines specifically calls for the testing of replication-competent status of retroviruses intended

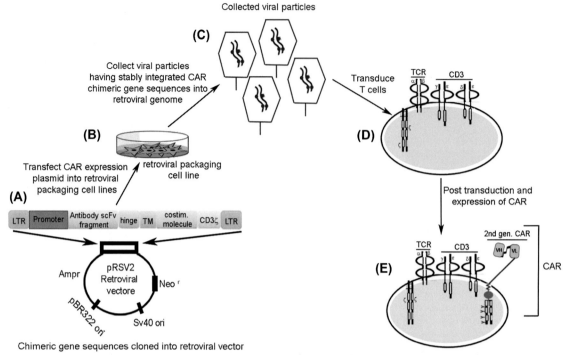

FIG. 3.4 Stepwise procedures involved in packaging of CAR-retroviral particles that can be used to infect T cells to express CARs. The first step in CAR-T production is cloning of CAR chimeric gene sequences into vector plasmids usually retroviral-based vectors **(A)**. The next step involves transfecting CAR-retroviral plasmids into retroviral packaging cell lines to create a stable vector producer cell line **(B)**. Once virus is produced from the vector producer cell line, the virus is collected, and titer determined. Viral supernatants can be stored in −80 for long-term storage or directly applied to infect host cells, for example, human T cells **(C)**. T cells are subsequently infected with CAR-viral supernatants, the transduction efficiency and percent modification of T cell with CARs will depend up on the MOI of the virus produced **(D-E)**.

to apply for modifying T cells [25], which is due to the fact that after T cells are virally transduced, the chimeric gene products are expressed on primary cells, a final product that may be delivered to the patients. Technically, the percentage of CAR T-cell modification depends on the quality of the vectors used to produce virus in helper cells. The two types of retroviral-based vector systems have found wider application in CAR therapy. These include γ-retroviruses and lentiviruses, and both seem to have performed very well in achieving an optimal modification of T cells in the in vitro settings and in clinical trials.

Integrating γ-retroviruses and lentiviral-based vectors have been predominantly used to clone chimeric genes for CAR production and subsequent infection of primary T cells for preclinical and clinical applications. The CAR cloning vectors have undergone extensive molecular modifications, and employ enhanced biosafety features since the first retroviral expression vector

pRSV2-neo and pRSV3-gpt was used to clone chimeric Ig (V_L and V_H)-TCR ($C\alpha$ and $C\beta$) genes in mice [26] (Fig. 3.5A,B). The pRSV2-neo and pRSV3-gpt contain long terminal repeats (LTR) derived from Rous sarcoma virus 3'LTR (DNAX Research Institute).

The sophisticated technical improvements in retroviral transduction methods and tailoring of retroviral vector LTR promoter sequences (that we will learn in the next sections) have greatly minimized the chances of production of replication-competent viruses inside the host cells [27]. Nevertheless, the lentiviral-based CAR vectors offer better choice. The advantage of lentiviruses over γ-retroviruses is that they can infect nondividing cells and the chances of insertional mutagenesis may be minimal, which provides threefold advantages over γ-retroviruses: (1) the HIV-1 lentiviruses in addition to *gag-pol* and *env* genes that are common to all retroviruses contain two regulatory genes *tat* and *rev*, and four accessory genes *vpr*, *nef*, *vpu*, and *vif*. The

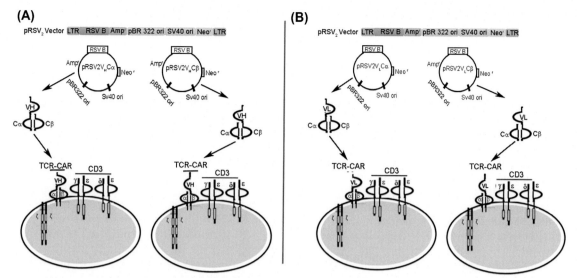

FIG. 3.5 Production of T-cell receptor (TcR) CAR. The first ever CAR was created by replacing TcRα and TcRβ variable domains with anti-2,4,6-trinitrophenyl (TNP) antibody variable heavy and light chain domains fused to constant domains of TcRα and TcRβ. Anti-2,4,6-trinitrophenyl (TNP) antibody variable heavy **(A)** and Anti-2,4,6-trinitrophenyl (TNP) antibody variable light chain genes **(B)** were cloned in retroviral expression vector pRSV2-neo. The pRSV2- contains LTR derived from Rous sarcoma virus 3′LTR. The homologous recombination enabled swapping of TcRα and TcRβ variable domains with anti-TNP variable domains.

tat and *rev* genes are essential for viral replications inside cells as well as gene transcription [28,29]. The *vpr, nef, vpu,* and especially *vif* genes have a crucial role in viral replication and virulence in vivo [30]. These HIV accessory and regulatory genes can offer additional control and biosafety features required for the expression of CARs in vivo and avoiding production of replication-competent retrovirus. For example, a vector system was created in which four accessory genes, *vpr, nef, vpu, vif,* and a virulence *env* genes of HIV-1 were deleted and pseudotyped with VSV-G protein. This strategy did not compromise the viral transduction to nondividing primary cells including lymphocytes, but provided an additional safety feature in terms of reducing the possibility of production of virulent HIV-1 particles inside the cells due to accessory and *env* gene deletions, thus, demonstrating the utility for human gene therapy [31]. In addition, several other safety features have been employed in HIV-1-based lentiviral vectors including a large deletion in the 3′LTR promoter of the vector construct that also deletes the TATA box. This self-inactivating vector construct improves the biosafety level significantly without compromising titer production and transgene expression [32]. (2) the lentiviral-based CAR vector system can be used to successfully transduce nondividing cells as much as dividing cells and can establish stable long-term expression of the CAR transgene. The fact that lentiviral-based CARs can achieve transduction in vivo in nondividing cells can dramatically enhance the scope of the CAR therapy to include target tissues as diverse as the brain, muscle, retina, liver etc. [33–35]. (3) the lentiviral LTRs tend to insert away from promoter regions of the genome minimizing the chances of insertional mutagenesis [36] in sharp contrasts with the γ-retrovirus LTR's that favor integration close to proto-oncogenes and enhancers risking the activation of oncogenes [37]. For example, the adverse effects were reported with the use of defective Moloney murine leukemia virus-based vectors in clinical trials involving children with X-linked severe combined immunodeficiency that leads to T-cell leukemia due to activation of proto-oncogene LMO-2 [38–40]. Similarly, gene therapy applied to chronic granulomatous patients lead to myelodysplasia and genomic instability [40]. Even though no notable adverse effects related to insertional mutagenesis have been reported using γ-retroviral-based vectors in humans [41], the production of replication-competent virus inside the host cells remains a concern. Moreover, the efforts to minimize such risk has been deliberated at various levels and covered under the institutional and federal guidelines. In the following sections, we will discuss in detail the retroviral vectors employed in the CAR production.

Retroviral Packaging System for CAR Production

The CAR sequences are cloned in retroviral-based vectors containing defective LTR promoters. That allows CAR chimeric gene sequences to be packaged as replication-deficient viruses without compromising infectivity (tropism). Several cell lines have been used for virus production. These packaging cell lines are transfected with combination of plasmids including the CAR expression plasmids and the plasmids containing virus assembly components flanked by the separate promoters and LTRs. These plasmids are collectively referred to as transfer plasmids.

The γ-retroviruses assembly components include *gag-pol* and *env* genes. *Gag* (Group Antigens) encodes core viral structural proteins, RNA genomic-binding proteins, and nucleoprotein core complex, *Pol* encodes reverse transcriptase (please refer to Fig. 3.7). The reverse transcriptase enzyme performs the reverse transcription of genomic RNA into cDNA that eventually forms a double stranded retroviral DNA provirus. The end sequences of *Pol* gene also encode RNA integrase (IN) that mediates integration of retroviral DNA into host genome [42,43]. The *env* gene encodes viral envelope protein. The most common *env* gene is VSV-G, which is used across γ-retroviruses and lentivirus-based vectors. Another commonly used envelope protein for retroviral gene transfer to human cells is RD114 derived from feline endogenous virus [44]. The *env* genes can be used to pseudotype viruses to alter virus tropism allowing viruses to infect a wide range of cells. The LTRs and *gag-pol-env* isoforms of γ-retroviruses and lentiviruses are not interchangeable.

Finally, the chimeric sequences of CARs are cloned into transfer plasmids (Fig. 3.6A,B). The common transfer plasmids used in CAR therapy are derived from Moloney Murine Leukemia Viruses or are HIV based. The choice of cell lines used to package viruses depend on the choice of primary cells to be infected for clinical or preclinical applications. For example, HEK 293T cells provide greatest flexibility for virus tropism and is very optimal for in vitro experiments. As, all the components of retroviral packaging including the *Env* gene and transfer plasmids are ectopically expressed through various transfection protocols [45] (Fig. 3.6A). Phoenix-Eco or Phoenix-AMPHO, amphotropic packaging cell lines, PA317 (ATCC), FLYRD18 [46], and PG13 (ATCC) are the other commonly used CAR packaging cell lines for the in vitro production of CARs for preclinical applications as well as for the clinical grade CAR production (Fig. 3.6B). The second-generation phoenix cell lines first developed by the Gary Nolan at Stanford University are referred to as helper free retroviral packaging cell lines because *Gag-Pol* and/or *Env* genes have been stably expressed in these cell lines, thus, eliminating the need to ectopically express these plasmids [47–49]. If the phoenix cell lines have *Env* gene stably expressed, the virus tropism cannot be altered. However, if the *Env* gene is not stably expressed and needed to be ectopically transfected then virus tropism can be altered. The Pheonix-ECO expresses viral envelope gene designed to target mouse and rat cells, whereas

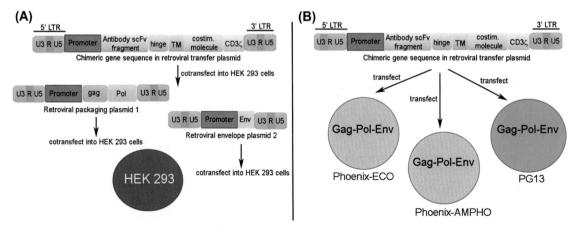

FIG. 3.6 Production of high-titer CAR retroviruses through utilizing transient transfection methods, for example, HEK 293 cell lines **(A)** or using producer cell lines, for example, Phoenix-ECO, Phoenix-AMPHO, or PG13 packaging lines **(B)**. Utilizing HEK 293 as a packaging cell line comes with an advantage of controlling virus tropism through pseudotyping of retroviral virions with ectopic expression of the viral envelope genes such as gibbon ape leukemia virus gene (GaLV) or vesicular stomatitis virus (VSV-G).

Phoenix-AMPHO have been designed to target mammalian cells including human cells https://web.stanford.edu/group/nolan/_OldWebsite/retroviral_systems/retsys.html. Similarly, PG13 retroviral packaging cell line, which is derived from mouse cell line, can be pseudotyped to target human cells [20].

The γ-retrovirus or lentivirus-based vector constructs containing chimeric gene sequences upon transfection into the host ecotrophic or amphotropic cell lines transcribe RNA transcripts. If the CAR expression vectors are transfected transiently into packaging cell lines, for example, PG13 cell line (PG13 cell line is derived from TK-NIH3T3 mouse cells expressing Gibbon ape leukemia virus genes), the CAR retroviral production will be transient requiring new transfections each time to produce fresh viruses. Therefore, a stable CAR expressing packaging cell lines can be very useful. For example, to generate high-titer-producing cell line clones stably expressing CARs for human T-cell infections, the CAR expression plasmid needs to be transfected into ecotrophic cell line, for example, Pheonix-ECO. The Pheonix-ECO will package and produce cell-free CAR vectors packaged as viruses that can infect mouse cell lines, for example, PG13. Subsequently, upon infecting PG13 cell line with cell-free vector stocks obtained with CAR transfection of Pheonix-ECO cell lines, the PG13 cell line will stably integrate CAR sequences into the genome that along with the *Gag-Pol* and/or *Env* genes can generate a stable vector producer cell line. The CAR expressing stable vector producer cell line may need to be subcloned by limiting dilution assays to select high-titer vector producer cells. The high-titer-producing cells may be selected using cell-sorting techniques.

The RNA transcripts in vector producer cell lines translate chimeric proteins that can be expressed on the packaging cell lines and also gets packaged and exported as virus particles containing chimeric genomic RNA transcripts including the viral reverse transcriptase and integrase enzymes. These are collected, stored, and used to infect target cells. The chimeric RNA transcripts are reverse transcribed inside the target T cells to form duplex DNA containing LTRs. The dsDNA sequences are bound by the integrase enzymes catalyze an integration reaction with host genome, which is mediated by the bound integrase [50,51]. Overall, an important step in the CAR expression is the integration of CAR DNA duplex into the genome of primary cells where the chances of producing additional viruses is minimal. Nevertheless, host primary cells are routinely tested for retroviral production.

The retroviral-based vectors have been extensively modified to be safer for human use. The most successful CAR developed to date, the CD19-CAR uses lentiviral or γ-retroviral-based vectors (transfer plasmids), the concern of insertional mutagenesis presented by the use of retroviruses have nevertheless persisted. Among the modifications introduced in retroviral vectors to reduce insertional mutagenesis includes deleting U3 sequences in the 3′ LTR. That potentially prevents the U3 of 3′LTR from serving as promoter in case U3 of 5′LTR becomes disrupted in the cells as that could lead to the retroviral oncogenesis [52] (Fig. 3.7). In addition, replacing lentiviral U3 promoter in the 5′LTR with truncated cytomegalovirus (CMV) enhancer/TATA promoter elements has reduced the risk of insertional mutagenesis without significantly affecting infectivity and titer production [53]. Nevertheless, several nonintegrating lentiviral vectors (NILVs) have recently been developed. HIV-based lentiviral vectors hold immense potential to be used in gene therapy especially due to their capacity to integrate nonspecifically into host genome and infectivity of nondividing cells.

Yet, LV vectors similar to γ-retroviruses have potential to cause insertional mutagenesis due to nonspecific integration if occur close to oncogene or tumor suppressor genes. Lentivirus integrase (IN) is one crucial 32 kd enzyme needed for transgene integration into host genome. Integrase is encoded by the *Pol* gene and binds within the U3 and U5 (ATT) DNA sequences in the LTRs to catalyze viral DNA integration into the

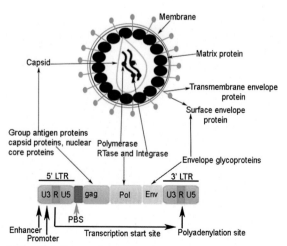

FIG. 3.7 Shows the genes that encode retroviral core structure as well as viral genomic core.

host genome [54]. Therefore, to develop HIV1 lentivirus-based NILVs, point mutations are introduced in the integrase enzyme that causes vectors to be defective specifically in integration but retains reverse transcription capacity [55]. NILVs due to their lack of integration with the host genome accumulate in the nucleus as naked linear DNA that may undergo circularization due to recombination between DNA LTRs followed by ligation of the DNA ends and are able to express CAR transgene. However, these circular DNA NILVs dilute out with the mitosis and CAR expression can be lost from the cells [56,57]. Therefore, for the stable CAR expression, NILV plasmids have been modified to include gene sequences of scaffold/matrix attachment region (S/MAR). The S/MAR is composed of genomic DNA sequences that anchor chromatin with the nuclear matrix protein by binding to scaffold attachment factor protein A (SAF-A). Therefore, during mitotic divisions, S/MAR allows NILV plasmids to be attached to the nuclear matrix preventing dilution of CARs [58,59]. The potential of NILV-based CARs for the CAR therapy has not been extensively tested. However, the technology certainly holds promise especially with added safeguards against insertional mutagenesis.

Transposon-Based System for CAR Cloning and Expression

A new genetic engineering technology known as *sleeping beauty (SB)* [60,61] and *PiggyBac* [62] is becoming popular for clinical grade CAR production primarily due to their potential to deliver an efficient, safer, and stable CAR expression [63]. Moreover, SB and PiggyBac system can accommodate large sizes of the transgene (Cargo DNA). In SB system, a CAR expression cassette (cargo DNA) are cloned in transposon-based vectors such as *pSBSO* flanked by inverted repeat/direct repeat (IR/DR) sequences driven by EF-1α/HTLV. In addition, a second expression plasmid such as CMV-driven SB-11 (pCMV-SB11) that encodes transposase is also used. The transposase recognizes IR/DR sequences and mediates precise integration of transposon into a TA dinucleotide sequences in the genome. The transposon-CAR expression cassette and transposase expression plasmids can be electroporated into primary T cells using nucleofector technology (Lonza). Finally, primary T cells expressing CARs can be activated ex vivo using artificial antigen-presenting cells (aAPC) such as γ-irradiated aK562—erythroleukemic cell line that can be ectopically transfected to express cognate tumor antigen (Fig. 3.8). A very useful protocol designed by Davidson

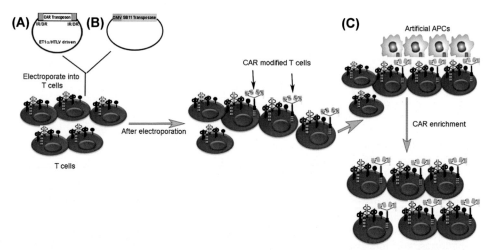

FIG. 3.8 Sleeping beauty (SB) system. In SB system, a CAR expression cassette is cloned in transposon-based vectors such as *pSBSO* flanked by inverted repeat/direct repeat (IR/DR) sequences, which is driven by EF-1α/HTLV **(A)**. A second expression plasmid CMV-driven SB-11 (pCMV-SB11) that encodes transposase is also used **(B)**. The two plasmids *pSBSO* and pCMV-SB11 are transfected into T cells. The transposase recognizes IR/DR sequences and mediates precise integration of transposon into a TA dinucleotide sequence in the genome. The transposon-CAR expression cassette and transposase expression plasmids can be electroporated into primary T cells using nucleofector technology. Finally, CAR expressing primary cells can be activated ex vivo using artificial antigen-presenting cells (aAPC) such as γ-irradiated aK562—erythroleukemic cell lines expressing cognate tumor antigen **(C)**.

et al. describes the procedure of using SB transposon system for stable gene expression in mouse embryonic stem cells [64].

The *PiggyBac* system consists of a *PiggyBac* vector and *Super PiggyBac transposase*. The Super PiggyBac transposase recognizes inverted terminal repeat (ITR) sequences and integrates ITRs and intervening chimeric gene sequences (Cargo DNA) into TTAA sites in the genome. Similar to SB system, *Super PiggyBac transposase* expression vector and *PiggyBac* vector can be cotransfected using electroporation method. One of the key advantages with the *PiggyBac* system is that the transgene along with the ITR can be excised from the genome using the excision only PiggyBac transposase. Therefore, control on shutting on and off CAR expression in PiggyBac system could help avoiding off-target cytotoxicity and cytokine storm syndrome observed with some CARs. The System Biosciences company specializes in creating PiggyBac system-based vectors and other gene therapy resources https://www.systembio.com/.

VECTORS USED FOR CAR PRODUCTION

This section will provide the list of vectors that have been used to clone CAR transgenes for targeting murine and human cells for in vitro and in vivo studies as well as in some selected clinical trials. Predominantly and successfully, it has been the retroviral vectors that have been used in CAR cloning and for targeting human and murine T cells. Some of these vectors have also been used in clinical applications. Lately, the lentiviral-based vectors have been extensively applied in clinical trials with the CARs. These include the third-generation self-inactivating lentiviral vector plasmids, pRRL-SIN-CMV-eGFP-WPRE (Cell Genesys, San Francisco, CA) that have been used successfully to target CD19$^+$ B-cell cancers in the clinical trials involving refractory chronic lymphocyte leukemia (NCT01029366) [65,66]. Moreover, the same vector system has also been used in studies involving immunodeficient mouse xenograft model of pre-B-cell acute lymphoblastic leukemia [67]. The pRRL-SIN-CMV-eGFP-WPRE lentiviral vector has been used to clone antimesothelin CARs (mesoCAR-T cells) containing 4I-BB costimulatory molecule and CD3ζ signaling domain to target mesothelin surface protein. In one such study, mesoCAR-T cells successfully eradicated mesothelioma xenograft tumors in NSG mice [68]. It is important to note that lentiviral-based CAR production is usually achieved with combination of three plasmids [31]: (1) The CAR-containing transfer plasmid, for example, pRRL-SIN-CMV-eGFP-WPRE [67]. (2) The packaging construct, for example,

pCMVΔR8.91 expressing *Gag, Pol, Tat,* and *Rev.* (3) The envelope plasmid, for example, pMD.G. Vectors can be engineered for in vitro and in vivo application with all three plasmids required to be transfected into 293T cells [33]. Similarly, the pCDH lentiviral plasmid was used to clone CEA to target CEA$^+$ colorectal cancers (CRC) in phase I clinical trial (NCT02349724) [69]. Some of the commonly used retroviral vectors include MSGV (mouse stem cell virus-based splice gag vector). The MSGV vector was used to clone anti-CD19 scFv second-generation CAR in the phase 1 dose-escalation trial involving children and young adults with acute lymphoblastic leukemia (NCT01593696) [70,71]. The SFG-retroviral vector was used to clone humanized rat antihuman scFv-CD33 and scFv 123 CAR to target NSG mice implanted with primary AML cells and AML cell line (KG1) expressing myeloid antigens CD33 and CD123 [72]. Moreover, the SFG-retroviral vector was used to clone MUC1-specific third-generation CAR containing CD28 and OX40 costimulatory domains and CD3ζ signaling domain. The MUC1 CAR demonstrated eradication of MUC1$^+$ tumor cell lines in vitro as well as in the in vivo xenograft tumor mouse model engrafted with MUC1 expressing MDA-MB-435 cells [73]. The SFG retroviral vector has also been used to produce first-generation HER2 CAR to eradicate medulloblastoma cell lines and primary tumors ex vivo as well as xenograft tumors in immunodeficient mice [74]. Similarly, a second-generation HER2-CAR containing CD28 costimulatory domain and CD3ζ signaling domain was cloned into SFG retroviral vectors and tested in a phase I/II clinical study (NCT00902044) involving recurrent/treatment refractory HER$^+$ sarcoma patients [75]. The SFG retroviral was also used to clone PSMA-specific scFv fused with CD28 and TCRζ [76]. PSMA is a glutamate carboxypeptidase membrane protein expressed on normal prostate epithelial cells but is over expressed in prostrate carcinoma [77]. The LXSN retroviral vector contains MuLV LTRs and a neomycin resistance gene under the control of SV40 promoter. The LXSN vector was used to clone mouse anti-G250 scFv first-generation CAR to target mouse renal cell carcinoma antigen. The G250 CAR utilizes signaling domain derived from gamma (γ-chain) of FcεRI present on mast cells [78]. The MFG vectors that carry Mo-MuLV LTRs were used for cloning bispecific anti-CEA-CAR to target CEA$^+$ liver metastasis in a phase I clinical trial (NCT01373047, RWH 11-335-99) [79]. Moreover, the same vector system was also used for the transmission of human genes such as *β-globin* and immune modulator GM-CSF [80,81] as well as for the in vivo transduction of IL2 and IL4 genes into metastasized tumors [82]. The MFG retroviral vector with Mo-MuLV LTRs plus neomycin phosphotransferase gene (*neo*) was used to clone first-generation MOv-γ CAR. The scFv was derived from Mov18 monoclonal antibody. The MOv-γ CAR contains the γ-signaling domain derived from Fc receptor γ-chain [83]. The MOv-γ CAR has been tested in vitro, in vivo in mice studies as well as clinically in a phase I study involving metastatic ovarian cancer [84–86]. The rkat43.2 retroviral vector was used to clone CC49-z TAG72 chimeric antigen receptor to target TAG72 in a clinical trial involving patients with metastatic CRC [87,88]. TAG72 is a mucin antigen expressed by the adenocarcinoma. The pMP71 retroviral vector was also used for cloning first-generation anti-CEA CAR (MFEζ) to target CEA$^+$ tumors in phase I/II clinical trial [(NCT 01212887), EUDRACT-2005-004085-16] [89]. The pLXSN retroviral vector was used to clone mouse-specific anti-CEA scFv second-generation CAR to target mouse CEA$^+$ pancreatic adenocarcinoma cells engrafted into the pancreas of CEA transgenic mice [90].

PROTOCOL FOR CAR PRODUCTION IN LABORATORY SETTINGS FOR PRECLINICAL APPLICATIONS

Various generations of CARs (as discussed in Chapter 2) have been created to improve antitumor efficacy [26,91–93]. A first-generation CAR-modified T cells have shown limited antitumor cytotoxicity in vivo and have been shown to undergo activation-induced cell death. The second-generation CARs apart from containing antigen-binding scFv domain (signal-1) also incorporates costimulatory CD28 or 4I-BB costimulatory molecule (signal-2) [94]. The incorporation of costimulatory signal-2 have rendered CAR modified T cells resistant to activation-induced cell death, promoted type I cytokine production, and provide prolonged antitumor effect in vivo [92,95,96]. The third-generation CARs incorporate two costimulatory molecules [97]. The advantages of incorporating two costimulatory molecules in CAR design are still being evaluated. However, the overall expectations with third-generation CARs is that they will improve antitumor activity against solid cancers.

Achieving an optimal CAR modification of T cells can be challenging. The poor ex vivo expansion of patient-derived T cells can impose significant hindrances. Traditionally, OKT3 has been employed to activate T cells before viral transduction step; however, that does not improve the percent modification of T cells significantly. To overcome these limitations, a powerful new technology that develops clinical grade CD3/CD28 beads for ex vivo activation and expansion of human T cells is expected to have huge clinical application especially for immunotherapy applications [98,99]. The CD3/CD28 dynabeads produced by the Thermo Fisher can produce 100- to 1000-fold expansion of T cells in a relatively shorter time frame. Furthermore, studies have already established the utility of this technology while working with large sample sizes [100].

Keeping in consideration these emerging new technologies, we provide herein three protocols. Protocols 1 and 2 have been tested and standardized with third-generation CARs combined with CD3/CD28-mediated activation of T cells. In contrast, protocol 3 has been tested and standardized with γ-retroviral-based second-generation CARs combined with OKT3-mediated activation. OKT3-mediated activation and subsequent modification of T cells with CARs are still being used in the clinical and preclinical production of CARs. The protocols 1 and 2 can be applied with third-generation lentiviral vectors that may be modified to include fluorescent proteins, for example, mCherry red fluorescent proteins that can aid in sorting CAR-positive cells through flow cytometry allowing estimation of the percent modification of target cells less cumbersome. The protocols 1 and 2 have been specifically designed for preclinical testing of third-generation CARs with a view that future CARs especially those designed to target solid cancers will be heavily modified and may contain several accessory molecules in the design to redirect trafficking to tumor sites, for the delivery of cytokines, and self-destruction mechanisms to avoid autoimmunity.

Production of Third-Generation CAR Lentiviral Particles
Materials
Third-generation CAR vector: As discussed, a third-generation CAR incorporates humanized anti-scFv fused with a polypeptide linker, a hinge, two costimulatory molecules usually CD28 and 4-1BB, and CD3ζ signaling endodomains. In addition, third-generation CARs may be labeled with fluorescent proteins, for example, EGFP or mCherry at the C-terminus of CD3ζ. The advantage of having fluorescent protein in the CAR can allow straightforward determination of percent modification of T cells with CARs without need of staining with fluorochrome-conjugated antibodies.

Primary Human T cells: Heparinized peripheral blood can be obtained from healthy donors. CD4 and CD8 T cells can be isolated using the CD4, CD8 enrichment kits, for example, EasySep Human CD4$^+$ or CD8$^+$

T-Cell Enrichment Kit (STEMCELL Technologies). T cells can be cryopreserved in 90% heat-inactivated FBS and 10% DMSO.

Reagents for lentivirus production: For lentivirus production, the following reagents are needed: low passaged HEK293FT cells (Invitrogen), T175 flasks (e.g., Denville Scientific), and Ultraculture media (e.g., Lonza). The Ultraculture media is supplemented with 2 mM L-glutamine, 100U/mL penicillin, 100 μg/mL streptomycin, 1 mM sodium pyruvate, and 50 mM sodium butyrate. Human T-cell growth medium [e.g., AIM5 or X-Vivo 15 (Lonza)] supplemented with 10 mM N-acetyl L-Cysteine (Sigma—Aldrich), 5% Human AB serum (e.g., Valley Biomedical), 55 μM 2-mercaptoethanol (Thermo Scientific), and IL2 [50 IU/mL (Chiron or Prometheus)].

10PSGN media. The 10PSGN media is prepared with 10% FBS and supplemented with 1X Pen/Strep, 1X Glutamine, 1X Sodium Pyruvate. The UPSGBN is made from Ultraculture media supplemented with 1X Pen/Strep, 1X Glutamine, 1X Sodium Butyrate, 1X Sodium Pyruvate. Polyethylenimine (PEI) (Sigma). NaCl: 0.15M filter sterilized. Sucrose (20%) filter sterilize. Retronectin (e.g., Clontech). Human T-activator beads, CD3/CD28 Dynabeads (Thermo Scientific). Non-TC treated six-well plates (e.g., Denville Scientific).

Plasmids for lentiviral packaging system. The following viral packaging plasmids can be used: pMD2.G encoding VSV-G pseudotyped envelope protein (available from Addgene), pDelta 8.74 (available from Addgene), and pAdv (available from Promega). In addition, the pHR vector for transgene expression.

Equipment list: A cell culture incubator, Beckman ultracentrifuge, −80°C deep freezer, BSL2 certified hood, flow cytometer, automated cell counter, and centrifuges.

To begin the protocols, lentiviral particles need to be produced in sufficient quantity and stored. Therefore, provided herein first is the procedure that was used for CAR lentiviral production.

Actual procedure: All media required for the lentiviral production were prepared before beginning the procedure.

1. **Day 0:** A low passage HEK293FT cells were plated inside T175 flask in 20 mL of 10PSGN media.
2. **Day 1:** At 60%—80% confluency, HEK293FT cells were transfected with the combination of retroviral packaging plasmids, pDelta (vector contains gag pol tat rev genes), VSVG and transfer plasmid (third-generation CAR expression plasmid). Provided below is the transfection protocol for one reaction:

   a. PEI transfection reagent and 0.15M NaCl were briefly vortexed and warmed to room temperature before use.
   b. PEI master mix was prepared by adding 350 μL of PEI to 900 μL of 0.15 M NaCl.
   c. DNA plasmid mix was prepared by adding 1.25 mL of 0.15 M NaCl to a sterile tube. To the tube were added a 22 μg of viral plasmids in the following ratio: 15 (pDelta): 5 (VSV-G): 2 (pAdv; empty vector). To this was added 22 μg CAR expression plasmid, and vortexed briefly.
   d. To the (c) was added 1.25 mL of PEI mix prepared in (b). Total volume in the tube was maintained around 2.50 mL
   e. Plasmid master was incubated for 10 minutes at room temperature.
   f. During the 10 minutes incubation, cell culture media of HEK293FT cells was replaced and fresh 7.5 mL prewarmed 10PSGN media was added.
   g. The plasmid-PEI mix was gently added to the flasks. Moreover, the flask was swirled gently to allow the plasmid mix to spread evenly
   h. Flask was placed inside the incubator for 24 hours
3. **Day 2:** After 24 hours, the medium of the flask was replaced by adding 20 mL of prewarmed UPSGBN media without detaching the cells.
4. **Day 3:** Virus supernatant was collected in 50 mL falcon tubes on ice. 20 mL of fresh prewarmed UPSGBN media was added into the flask to collect more virus if needed.
5. The collected virus was spun to remove the cell debris, and supernatants were filter sterilized over Beckman ultracentrifuge tubes using 0.45 μm sterile filters. Filter-sterilized virus was stored at 4°C for immediate use. Moreover, for long-term storage, viral supernatant was stored in small aliquots in −80°C.

To determine if the third-generation CAR expression on CD4 or CD8 T cells can be improved with CD3/CD28 bead activation, the CD4$^+$ or CD8$^+$ T cells were enriched from the human PBMCS and stimulated for 48 hours with CD3/CD28 dynabeads. The cell-to-bead ratio was maintained at 1:3 in both protocols.

Protocol 1

1. Nontissue culture six-well plates were coated with retronectin for 2 hours at RT. After 2 hours, retronectin-coated plates were washed with PBS.
2. Before starting the transduction, the CD3/CD28 bead-activated T cells were taken out from the incubator and transferred into a falcon tube and

placed under the magnet to remove the beads. Subsequently, cells were counted and spun at 1500 RPM for 5 minutes, and an estimated 250×10^3 cells were used for the viral transduction as described in the following steps.

3. T cells prepared in the step-2 were suspended in 500 μL CAR viral supernatant diluted in 1.5 mL (1 : 4 dilution) of T-cell growth medium supplemented with 100 U/mL of IL2 and protamine sulfate (5 μg/mL). This 2 mL solution containing diluted virus and bead-activated T cells were transferred to the retronectin-coated plates. Plates were sealed, balanced, and spun at 2500 rpm for 2 hours at room temperature.

4. At the end of the spin, seals were removed, and plates were placed in 37°C incubator for 3-hour. After 3-hour incubation, plates were removed from the incubator and entire content in the wells was transferred to a falcon tube and spun for 5 minutes at room temperature. At the end of the spin, the supernatant was carefully aspirated and discarded. The cell pellet was suspended in a fresh diluted virus as described in step 3 and transferred back to the original retronectin-coated plates. Plates were sealed and subjected to second round of spin at 2500 rpm for 2 hours at room temperature.

5. After the end of the second spin, plate seal was removed, and plates were placed back into the incubator for additional 3 hours.

6. After three-hour incubation time, plates were removed from the incubator and without any additional spin, fresh 2-mL medium containing 100 U/mL of IL2 was added and placed back in the 37°C incubator. After 48-hour incubation, cells were subjected to the flow cytometry analysis to determine the CAR expression through fluorophore detection.

The data obtained from protocol 1 using the bead activation revealed on average 40% CAR-positive T cells compared to the unactivated control, which is significant improvement over the unactivated controls.

Protocol 2

In the protocol 2, we performed a virus concentration step before the actual transduction of CD3/CD28 bead-activated CD4 T cells. The virus concentration protocol is described in the following steps.

Virus concentration:

1. The freshly collected virus supernatants were filter sterilized over Beckman ultracentrifuge tubes using 0.45-μm sterile filters. A 50-mL virus supernatant was used for the concentration procedure.

2. 2 mL of filter-sterilized 20% sucrose was subsequently added gently to a tube containing 50-mL filter-sterilized virus.

3. Tubes were subjected to ultracentrifugation using sterilized SW28 rotor at 22,000 rpm at 4°C for 2 hours.

4. After the end of the spin, tubes were placed in ice. Supernatants were carefully aspirate off without disturbing the viral pellet.

5. To the viral pellet (depending upon the size) were added carefully between 300 and 500 μL of cell growth medium by taking pipette close to the pellet settled at the bottom of the tube. Pellet in PBS were left unperturbed for 2 hours at 4°C. After two-hours, virus pellet was gently suspended in PBS using the pipette and avoiding the bubbles. Virus aliquots were transferred into sterilized Eppendorf tubes.

6. For immediate use, viral aliquots were stored at 4°C. Moreover, for long-term storage, virus aliquots were transferred to −80°C.

Virus transduction:

1. Before performing the actual virus transduction procedure, we used the concentrated virus as prepared earlier. The nontissue culture six-well plate was treated with retronectin at the concentration of 32 μg/mL. Coated plates were incubated for 2 hours at room temperature.

2. After two-hour incubation, retronectin solution was aspirated off, and the plate was blocked for 30 minutes with 2 mL blocking solution (2% BSA dissolved in 1x PBS) at the room temperature.

3. Plates were washed with 1x PBS.

4. A 3.5 mL of concentrated CAR virus was transferred into retronectin-coated plate.

5. Plate was sealed and spun at 1200xg for 1 hour and 30 min.

   During the spin, the CD3/CD28 bead-activated T cells—maintained at 1:3 cell and bead ratio and activated for 48 hours—were removed from the incubator. Cells were transferred into falcon tube and placed under the magnet to remove beads. The cells were counted and approximately 250,000 cells/mL were suspended in T-cell growth media supplemented with 100 U/mL of IL2.

6. After the end of the spin, viral supernatant was aspirated off from the retronectin-coated plate.

7. The bead-activated T cells at the concentration of ∿250,000 cells/mL were transferred into the retronectin-coated plate and spun at 1200xg for 1 hour with a reduced breaking speed (deceleration = 3).

8. Following the spin, plates were transferred into incubator (maintained at 37°C and 5% CO_2 level).
9. Cells were analyzed for CAR expression at 48-hour posttransduction.

The results commonly obtained from protocol 2 demonstrated that T cells modified with CAR can achieve up to ∿70% modification, which is a twofold improvement over the protocol 1. In addition, the median fluorescent intensity (MFI) values can be significantly improved.

Protocol 3

The protocol 3 is provided that can be used to transduce T cells with γ-retrovirus-based first- and second-generation CAR vectors.

Day 0

The blood filters or blood collars can be obtained from blood banks and subject to Ficoll density gradient elutriation to isolate PBMCs. The PBMC's at 2×10^6/mL density are cultured in cell culture flasks in AIM-V media with 5% heat inactivated human serum. Cells are activated with OKT3 (50 μg/mL)-mediated activation in the presence of IL2 (300 IU/mL) for 48 hours.

Day 2

Procedure coating the plates. The six-well nontissue culture plates are used for the transduction.
1. Coat the wells with a retronectin solution.
2. Prepare the retronectin solution as follows. Add 10 μg/mL of retronectin solution in 1 mL 1x PBS buffer. Pipette 1 mL of solution into each well and shake the plate to cover the entire well bottom with the solution.
Store at 4°C overnight.

Day 3

Prepare viral supernatants. The CAR retroviral vector supernatants with predetermined titer and transduction unit values are stored in −80°C freezer.
1. Take out the frozen viral supernatant vials out from the −80°C freezer and thaw on ice or at 4°C
2. Warm the AIM-V media supplemented with 5% human serum and IL2 (300 IU/mL). In addition, thaw the protamine sulfate vial (which is usually stored at −20°C freezer).
3. If needed, dilute the viral supernatant with AIM5 complete media and bring the volume to 2 mL.
4. To the 1-mL viral aliquot, add 1 mL complete media plus 1 μg/mL protamine sulfate.

5. Take out the T cells from the 37°C incubator, count the cells, and transfer 10×10^6 cells in a falcon tube and spin at 400 g for 10 minutes.
6. After the spin, discard the supernatant and suspend T cells in 2-mL retroviral supernatant solution prepared in step 4.
7. Take out retronectin-coated six-well plate from the 4°C fridge, aspirate off the retronectin solution, and wash two times with 1x PBS solution.
8. Transfer 2 mL retroviral solution to retronectin-coated six-well plate, seal the plate with paraffin-wrap, and spin at 2500 rpm for 90 minutes.
9. Gently take the plates out from centrifuge, remove the paraffin seal, and place the plate in 37°C cell culture incubator for 3 hours.
10. After the completion of the first 3-hour incubation time, take plates out from incubator and transfer the retroviral solution (2 mL) in each well into a 15 mL centrifuge tube to spin at 5 minutes at 400 g. Discard the supernatant.
11. Use the second batch of fresh virus to infect T cells second time following the steps 4−8 as described earlier.
12. After the completion of second spin at 2500 rpm for 90 minutes, gently take out the plate from centrifuge, remove the paraffin seal, and place plate back in 37°C cell culture incubator for 3 hours.
13. After the completion of the second 3-hour incubation time, take plates out from incubator, and transfer the retroviral solution (2 mL) in each well into a 15 mL centrifuge tube to spin at 5 minutes at 400 g. Discard the supernatant.
14. Use the third batch of fresh virus to infect T cells third time following the steps 4−8 as described earlier.
15. After the completion of third three-hour incubation, take plates out from incubator, remove the paraffin seal, and add additional 2 mL complete media with IL2 (300 IU/mL). Incubate for 24 hours.
16. After 24-hour incubation, cells can be washed to remove the virus and incubated for additional 48 hours. After which, cells can be analyzed through flow cytometry to determine the percent CAR modification of T cells, MFI values, and other parameters.

Expansion of Primary T Cells and Generation of CAR-Modified T cells

Promising results have been obtained both in vitro and in vivo animal models with the third-generation CARs developed to target solid cancers such as ERBB2 expressing breast cancer [101,102]. In contrast to second- and third-generation CARs, in vitro studies using first-generation CAR-modified T cells have shown suboptimal effector cytokine production and suboptimal antitumor activities [96,103]. Overall, the third-generation CARs incorporating two costimulatory molecules seem to have provided better clinical outcome for lymphoma patients [104]. Whether the third-generation CARs developed to target solid cancers can also produce better clinical outcomes remains to be seen. However, for the promise of better clinical outcome in patients, solid preclinical data can be very valuable. A better expansion of primary T cells and optimal expression of third-generation CARs can be essential for obtaining solid preclinical data and evaluating the antitumor responses. Subjecting human T cells before virus transduction protocols to two signal (signal 1 + 2) activation utilizing dynabeads may be essential for enhancing viral transduction efficiency as dynabead-mediated signal 1 + 2 activation leads to a greater proliferation rate compared to conventional OKT3 activation. Dynabeads are covalently linked with CD3 and CD28 monoclonal antibodies. Therefore, dynabeads essentially mimic in vivo antigen-presenting cells. In our experiments, we have achieved an effective expansion of CD4 T cells using CD3/CD28 beads in consistent with the results obtained by Li Y et al. [105]. An additional advantage of bead activation of T cells is an improvement in the CAR expression [106]. Several biotech companies such as Invitrogen and Miltenyi produce clinal grade CD3/CD28 activation reagents for the ex vivo expansion of T cells. These reagents include CTS CD3/28 Dynabeads, the Miltenyi MACS GMP ExpAct Treg beads, and Miltenyi MACS GMP TransAct CD3/28 beads [107]. As results have demonstrated that ex vivo expansion of primary T cells with beads can be much more efficient and permissive for CAR expression, a better CAR expression and antitumor responses can be anticipated for patient-derived T cells. Whether the T cells using clinical grade bead activation and expressing higher percentage of third-generation CARs can translate into better clinical response remains to be seen. It is not unconceivable that combining the improved expression of CARs on T cells followed by better ex vivo expansion can help scaling up the production of CAR T cells for clinical use. However, a high expressing CAR-modified T cells designed to target tumor-associated antigens on solid tumors may be associated with a pitfall of on-target/off-tumor toxicities. Therefore, a carefully controlled and extensive preclinical evaluation of such CARs must be performed before moving to actual clinical use.

In Vitro Testing of CAR-T Cells

Once T-cell receptors have been modified in 70% to 80% range with CARs, for example, second-generation anti-CEA-CAR or third-generation anti-HER2-CAR. The next step is the preclinical evaluation of CAR-T cells in the in vitro and in vivo experiments to evaluate their effector functions including the tumor-killing activities, effector cytokine production, expansion, and in vivo persistence. These properties are important to evaluate experimentally before CAR-T cells can be tested clinically in human patients. Achieving optimal percent modification of T cells with CARs is vital first step for the preclinical testing of CAR-T cells. As discussed in previous sections, traditionally OKT3 supplemented with IL2 have been utilized to activate T cells before subjecting them to CAR-retroviral vector infection cycles to modify their receptors. Lately, however, in the clinical settings while working with patient-derived T cells, CD3/CD28 bead-mediated activation have resulted much higher proliferation rates and higher percentage of CAR modification of T cells. Therefore, apart from OKT3, the CD3/CD28 bead-mediated activation is increasingly being employed to activate T cells before subjecting them to retroviral infection for CAR expression. Once T cells have been modified with CARs, the next step is determining their percentage modification and MFI values, which is usually evaluated through flow cytometry-based techniques. However, to determine the percentage of CAR-modified T cells comes with a caveat, which is the need to design an anti-scFv-specific fluorochrome-conjugated antiidiotype antibody to accurately assess the percent modification (Fig. 3.9A). Usually, anti-idiotype antibodies can be obtained in collaboration with the companies specializing in antibody production or generated in private labs. Interestingly, there is another way to bypass the requirement for anti-idiotype antibodies, which is cloning a fluorescent gene and inserting infrane with other chimeric gene sequences, for example, mCherry red-emitting fluorescent protein [108] (Fig. 3.9B). The monomeric mCherry is derived from *mRFP1* through introducing mutations that makes mCherry suitable for flow cytometry-mediated detection [109]. The *RFP1* is derived from coral genus *Discosoma* sp. The mCherry can be excited with yellow-green laser (561 nm) and can be detected in flow cytometry using the red filter (610/20 nm) [110,111]. Thus, bypassing the need to design an antiidiotype antibody in evaluating percent modification of CAR-T cells.

The next step in the in vitro characterization of CAR-T cells is testing their antitumor potency. The antitumor potency of CAR-T cells can be examined in coculture experiments using primary tumor cells or tumor cell lines

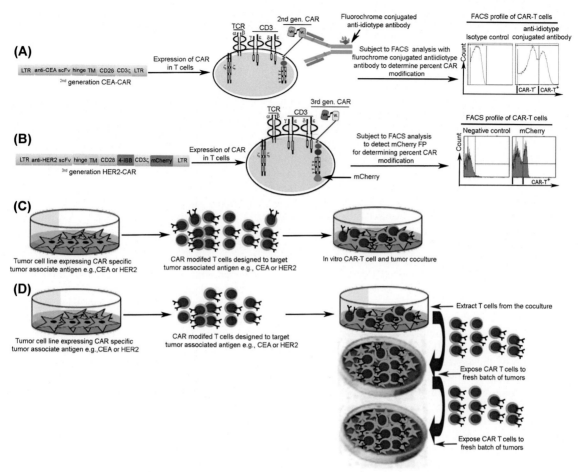

FIG. 3.9 The procedure by which CARs expressed on primary T cells can be identified and tested experimentally. **(A-B)** Chimeric gene sequences of second-generation anti-CEA CAR and third-generation anti-HER2 CAR. Note anti-HER2 CAR expresses fluorescent red-cherry gene. The CARs can be expressed stably or transiently in T cells. To determine the percentage modification of T cells, anti-idiotype fluorochrome-conjugated antibodies can be generated to detect anti-CEA CAR using flow cytometry method **(representative histogram, A)**. In contrast, anti-HER2 CAR expressing mCherry does not require generation of anti-idiotype antibody as fluorescent signal can be detected directly through flow cytometry method **(representative histogram, B)**. **(C)** Shows the procedure by which CARs can be tested for antitumor activity in the in vitro settings. CARs can be cocultured with tumor cell lines expressing cognate tumor-associated antigens then measuring CAR-mediated tumor lysis using various techniques, for example, chromium-51 release assay. **(D)** Demonstrates the procedure by which CAR antitumor potency can be tested in repeat coculture with tumor cell lines. Basically, CARs can be exposed to fresh batches of tumors repeatedly to demonstrate if CARs are able to lyse persistent tumors without losing potency.

expressing cognate tumor-associated antigen, for example, CEA tumor antigen expressing cells or HER2 expressing breast cancer cells (Fig. 3.9C). An important control for such experiments can be a tumor cell line that does not express the tumor antigen, for example, CEA^{-ve} or $HER2^{-ve}$ or the tumor cell line in which gene encoding the tumor antigen is knocked out. There are several parameters that must be taken into consideration before designing the CAR-T tumor coculture experiments. First, the tumor cell numbers must be adjusted with CAR T-cell numbers considering the percent modification of chimeric receptor. For example, if we are seeding one million tumor cells and plan to coculture these with one million CAR-T cells having

50% modification that implies we are setting 2:1 tumor and CAR-T ratio. However, if we are using T cells having 100% CAR modification (e.g., after cell sorting) with the equal number of the tumor cells in a coculture, we are setting a 1:1 ratio. It is essential that percent CAR modification of T cells is assessed through flow cytometry each time before performing tumor coculture experiment. Assessing the CAR-T expression also becomes essential as CAR transgene can be leaky and there have been reports of loss of CAR transgene expression in T cells [101]. Overall, in the tumor-killing assays, CAR T-cell ratio must always be maintained lower than tumor cell numbers because a single CAR-T cell can target multiple tumor cells. In addition, once a CAR-T cell makes a contact with the tumor cell, CAR-T cells can receive activation signals and such cells have huge potential to proliferate. Maintaining a lower CAR T-cell number in the tumor coculture is also important because in clinical settings patient-derived T cells may not achieve higher modification with CARs. Another important point to consider in CAR-T tumor coculture experiments is blocking the proliferation of metastatic tumor cells. The metastatic tumor cell lines such as MIP101 human colon carcinoma cancer cell line [112] or some of the breast cancer cell lines [113] have tremendous potential to proliferate. Therefore, to prevent extensive growth of tumor cell lines in cocultures, their proliferations must be stopped prior to coculture with CAR-T cells with the anticancer drugs such as Mitomycin C (Millipore, cat. 475820) etc. A failure to do so can significantly compromise the interpretation of the tumor-killing data.

Measuring tumor-killing activity

Several techniques are available that can aid in assaying and quantitation of immune cell-mediated cancer cytotoxicity. One of the classical techniques utilized by the labs is radioactive chromium-based chromium-51 release assay. The technique was developed more than 50 years ago by Brunner et al. [114]. In the chromium release assay, tumor cells expressing CAR-specific tumor antigens are radiolabeled with ^{51}Cr. The CAR-T cells (after taking into considering the percent modification) are incubated at different ratios with ^{51}Cr labeled tumor cells (usually E:T ratios may be in the ranges of 30:1, 10:1, 3:1, 1:1). The CAR-T tumor cells are incubated for 4 hours at 37°C. The percentage of specific tumor cell lysis is determined by measuring the ^{51}Cr release in the supernatant using liquid scintillation counter [115]. This technique can also help calculating the EC50 and EMax values that may be crucial in examining the CAR T-cell antigen-specific lysis. Apart from the ^{51}Cr

release assay, there are other non-radioactive fluorescent label-based techniques that can help quantitate tumor cell killings. For example, before coculture with the CAR-T cells, tumor cells can be transfected to almost 90% efficiency with a luciferase reporter, for example, renilla luciferase. That can be followed by their coculture with the CAR-T cells using different (E:T) ratio. The luciferase activity can be measured directly using a luminometer. Tests have confirmed that luciferase activity comes mostly from the live cells, thus, can help quantitating the overall tumor cell viability which can provide an indirect measure of percent tumor cell killings [116]. In addition, a lactate dehydrogenase release assay (Boehringer Mannheim) is also utilized for CTL-mediated tumor cytotoxicity assays [76].

Effector cytokine production. Another important measure of CAR-T cell effector functions is effector cytokine release such as IL2, IFNγ, and TNFα upon CAR-T contact with the tumor-associated antigens. Including costimulatory molecules such as CD28 and 4I-BB as signal 2 in the design of CARs have vastly improved effector cytokine release, proliferation, and in vivo persistence [117−120]. In contrast, the first-generation CARs that lack costimulatory molecules undergo aberrant activation-induced cell death and are poor producers of type I cytokines [96,121]. Therefore, it is essential to measure both cytokine release and tumor-killing activities side by side in the same experimental set-up. Because type I cytokines are released by the T cells, the supernatants saved from the CAR-T tumor coculture can be directly assessed for the cytokine production through ELISA or through internal staining techniques followed by flow cytometry based quantitation.

The effector cytokine release and tumor-killing activities must be measured in repeat cocultures including the tumor antigen negative cancer cells as controls. The idea is to test the persistence of CAR-T cells. For example, anti-CEA or anti-HER2 CAR T cells may be subjected to 48 hour coculture with CEA or HER2 antigen-rich malignant cancer cells and CEA^{-ve} or HER2^{-ve} control cancer cell lines. After which, anti-CEA or anti-HER2 CAR T cells may be recovered from coculture and exposed to a second and third batch of CEA or HER2 antigen-rich malignant cancer cells. The same procedure must be applied with the control tumor cells. The rationale for repeatedly exposing CAR T cells to fresh tumor targets can help assessing the persistence, tumor-killing capacity, and effector cytokine release against persistent tumor antigens that CAR-T cells are likely to be exposed in vivo (Fig. 3.9D).

In Vivo Testing of CAR-T Cells

CARs are designed to treat human cancers. Therefore, testing CAR-T cells in the in vivo model organisms for efficacy and toxicity studies could provide valuable data before moving to actual clinical trials. Unfortunately, up until now there has been no reliable model organism available that could be used to test human CAR-T cells. There are both ethical and technical limitations in that direction. For example, testing human CAR-T cells against human cancers in mouse model imposes several technical challenges. Take the example of commonly used immunodeficient nude mouse model. The nude mice are presented with spontaneous mutation ($Foxn1^{nu}$) (JAX stock #002019). The homozygous nude mutant mice are athymic and lacks T cells; however, other immune cells such as B cells and NK cells including the innate immune system are present [122,123]. The nude mice allows engraftment of human tumor cell lines. Moreover, as the mice lack hair the straightforward estimation of tumor growth can be performed. However, due to the presence of innate immune cells, human CAR T-cell engraftment that must be performed intravenously may be quickly rejected, and subsequent analysis related to tumor regression may not become possible to evaluate accurately. Some of the most important preclinical data expected to be obtained with the in vivo mice models includes CAR T-cell trafficking, in vivo persistence, type I cytokine release, and potential toxicities. However, with the innate immune system intact and partial loss of adaptive immune cells in nude mice, these critical data cannot be reliably obtained and interpreted. Therefore, nude mice model is not a good preclinical model to test human CAR-T cells antitumor activities. Similarly, the BALB/c-*scid* mice (JAX stock #001803) that possess severe combined immune deficiency spontaneous mutation $Prkdc^{scid}$, lack mature B and T cells but retain innate immunity. This mice strain is easy to engraft with xenograft tumors [124]; however, engrafting human CAR-T cells and subsequent antitumor activities imposes the similar limitations as with nude mice. One advantage, however, with this model is an adoptive transfer of modified T cells. The adoptive transfer of modified T cells can be performed using the syngeneic BALB/c donor that, however, would require to generate mouse-specific CAR-T cells. It is obvious that not many labs would be interested to generate mouse tumor-specific CAR-T cells. It is obvious from the discussion above that an in vivo mouse model that lack partially or completely both adaptive and innate immune system may serve the purpose of testing anticancer properties of human CAR-T cells. An ideal mouse model, therefore, can be one that apart from allowing human tumor cell lines or patient-derived xenograft tumor engraftment must also allow reconstitution of human hematopoietic system generating cells of both lymphoid and myeloid lineages such as B and T cells (lymphopoiesis), neutrophils, monocytes, dendritic cells (myelopoiesis), red blood cell, and platelets (erythropoiesis and megakaryopoiesis). The advantage of having functional human immune system reconstituted in mice will allow isolation and ex vivo modification of T cells with the CAR expression vectors. The CAR-modified T cells can be subsequently engrafted into human tumor xenograft recipient to evaluate antitumor effector functions. The nonobese diabetic/severe combined immunodeficient (NOD-*scid*) mice (Jackson stock # 001303)] may be one such mice model. The NOD.CB17 mice have *scid* spontaneous mutation $Prkdc^{scid}$. The NOD-*scid* lack mature T and B cells and reduced innate immune cells such as macrophages, NK, and dendritic cells and are also compliment deficient [125]. Studies have established that this mouse model can be engrafted with human xenograft tumors as well as human peripheral blood mononuclear cells [126]. However, whether this mouse model can be used for human CAR-T engraftment and can successfully generate CAR-T-mediated tumor killings need further studies. Another severely immunodeficient mouse model is NOD scid gamma mice commonly known as NSG mice (Jackson stock# 005557). The NOD mouse strain carries two mutations: *scid* and IL2 receptor γ-chain *(IL2-Rγ)* null mutations. The γ-chain of IL2 trimeric receptor is common among several cytokine receptors such as IL4, IL15, IL21, IL7, and IL9 [127]. The mutation in γ-chain in humans causes X-linked severe combined immunodeficiency. A complete T-cell defect is found in such patients. In contrast, the γ-chain null mutation in mice contributes to deficiency in number of cytokine receptor genes and disrupts cytokine receptor signaling pathways predominantly involving JAK-STAT signaling pathway leading to a severe deficiency in NK cells. In addition, NSG mice are deficient in innate immune system, presents with a defective complement system, defective macrophages, and have reduced dendritic cell numbers [128,129]. One of the unique features in NSG mice is that they can support human hematopoietic stem cell engraftment sustainable for more than 24 weeks. Ishikawa et al. demonstrated that NSG mice support hematopoiesis and lymphopoiesis upon engraftment of human CD34$^+$ stem cells or CD34$^+$CD38$^-$ cord blood cells that reconstituted human hematopoietic cells. That subsequently

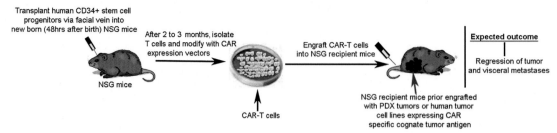

FIG. 3.10 Humanized NSG tumor mouse model that can be used to test CAR-T potency against human-derived patient xenograft tumors (PXT). To avoid interference from host innate immune system to the engrafted-xenograft tumors, human cord blood stem cells can be transplanted into irradiated newborn NSG mice to generate so-called humanized NSG mice. The humanized NSG mice is capable of reconstituting myelopoiesis as well as lymphopoiesis. After 2–3 months, T cells from adult reconstituted NSG mice may be isolated and subjected to retroviral transduction protocols to express a CAR, for example, anti-CD19 CAR. The anti-CD19 CAR can be subsequently injected back into hNSG mice pretransplanted with human tumors, for example, ALL leukemia cells expressing CD19 antigen. CAR-T cells in these mice can be evaluated for antitumor activity. The preclinical data obtained from such mice can prove very valuable for filing investigation new drug application and eventually for gaining approval from FDA to test CAR-T product in human patients.

differentiates into myeloid lineage cells (monocytes and dendritic cells), erythrocytes and megakaryocytes, and lymphoid lineage (T and B cells). The growth of innate and adaptive immune cells follows the lineage differentiation program through the common lymphocyte and myeloid progenitor cells [130]. The humanized NSG mice (human CD34$^+$ stem cell chimeras) can serve a best preclinical model to test CAR-T cells' antitumor activity as well as evaluating potential CAR-associated toxicities. These analyses become possible only because T cells from the humanized NSG mice can be modified with CARs and subsequently adoptively transferred into recipient NSG mice prior engrafted with the human tumor cells expressing cognate tumor antigens (Fig. 3.10).

If the tumor is successfully established and not rejected by the reconstituted innate and adoptive system in the NSG recipient mice. The CAR-T cells adoptively transferred into recipient mice can be reliably evaluated for the antitumor activity including effector cytokine release, in vivo CAR-T persistence at tumor sites as well as evaluating CAR-T-associated toxicities. One of the limitations with the NSG CAR-T model may be the number of CAR-T cells that could be engrafted. Relatively, a small number of CAR-T cells may be engrafted into NSG mice, and the optimal number may need to be tested experimentally for the objective interpretation of the actual data. Norelli et al. demonstrated the feasibility of the approach discussed above in evaluating human antigen-specific CAR-T-related toxicities. Norelli et al. transplanted human cord blood stem cells into irradiated newborn NSG mice to generate humanized NSG

mice capable of reconstituting myelopoiesis as well as lymphopoiesis. T cells in adult mice were subjected to express anti-CD19 and anti-CD44v6 CARs that were subsequently injected back into hNSG mice pre-transplanted with human chronic myeloid leukemia in lymphoid blast crisis ALL-CM leukemia cells expressing CD19 antigen whereas CD44v6 human myeloid leukemia antigen was stably expressed through lentiviral infection. CAR-T cells in these mice were able to perform antitumor activity normally but also recapitulated commonly reported CAR T-cell-related toxicities observed in humans such as cytokine-related syndrome and neurological events [131].

REFERENCES

[1] Nimmerjahn F, Ravetch JV. Fc-receptors as regulators of immunity. Adv Immunol 2007;96:179–204.

[2] Harwood PJ, Boden J, Pedley RB, Rawlins G, Rogers GT, Bagshawe KD. Comparative tumour localization of antibody fragments and intact IgG in nude mice bearing a CEA-producing human colon tumour xenograft. Eur J Cancer Clin Oncol 1985;21:1515–22.

[3] Bird RE, Hardman KD, Jacobson JW, Johnson S, Kaufman BM, Lee SM, et al. Single-chain antigen-binding proteins. Science 1988;242:423–6.

[4] Hariharan D, Saied A, Kocher HM. Analysis of mortality rates for pancreatic cancer across the world. HPB (Oxford) 2008;10:58–62.

[5] Nath S, Daneshvar K, Roy LD, Grover P, Kidiyoor A, Mosley L, et al. MUC1 induces drug resistance in pancreatic cancer cells via upregulation of multidrug resistance genes. Oncogenesis 2013;2:e51.

[6] Parkin DM. Global cancer statistics in the year 2000. Lancet Oncol 2001;2:533—43.

[7] O'Sullivan CC, Swain SM. Pertuzumab: evolving therapeutic strategies in the management of HER2-overexpressing breast cancer. Expert Opin Biol Ther 2013;13:779—90.

[8] Petkov VI, Miller DP, Howlader N, Gliner N, Howe W, Schussler N, et al. Breast-cancer-specific mortality in patients treated based on the 21-gene assay: a SEER population-based study. NPJ Breast Cancer 2016;2:16017.

[9] Howlader N, Morton LM, Feuer EJ, Besson C, Engels EA. Contributions of subtypes of non-hodgkin lymphoma to mortality trends. Cancer Epidemiol Biomarkers Prev 2016;25:174—9.

[10] Wang K, Wei G, Liu D. CD19: a biomarker for B cell development, lymphoma diagnosis and therapy. Exp Hematol Oncol 2012;1:36.

[11] Felder M, Kapur A, Gonzalez-Bosquet J, Horibata S, Heintz J, Albrecht R, et al. MUC16 (CA125): tumor biomarker to cancer therapy, a work in progress. Mol Cancer 2014;13:129.

[12] Miyake M, Taki T, Hitomi S, Hakomori S. Correlation of expression of H/Le(y)/Le(b) antigens with survival in patients with carcinoma of the lung. N Engl J Med 1992;327:14—8.

[13] Jakobovits A, Amado RG, Yang X, Roskos L, Schwab G. From XenoMouse technology to panitumumab, the first fully human antibody product from transgenic mice. Nat Biotechnol 2007;25:1134—43.

[14] Bruggemann M, Osborn MJ, Ma B, Buelow R. Strategies to obtain diverse and specific human monoclonal antibodies from transgenic animals. Transplantation 2017;101:1770—6.

[15] Lonberg N. Human antibodies from transgenic animals. Nat Biotechnol 2005;23:1117—25.

[16] Wege AK, Schmidt M, Ueberham E, Ponnath M, Ortmann O, Brockhoff G, et al. Co-transplantation of human hematopoietic stem cells and human breast cancer cells in NSG mice: a novel approach to generate tumor cell specific human antibodies. MAbs 2014;6:968—77.

[17] Yoshida S, Kobayashi T, Matsuoka H, Seki C, Gosnell WL, Chang SP, et al. T-cell activation and cytokine production via a bispecific single-chain antibody fragment targeted to blood-stage malaria parasites. Blood 2003;101:2300—6.

[18] Winter G, Griffiths AD, Hawkins RE, Hoogenboom HR. Making antibodies by phage display technology. Annu Rev Immunol 1994;12:433—55.

[19] Hammers CM, Stanley JR. Antibody phage display: technique and applications. J Invest Dermatol 2014;134:1—5.

[20] Miller AD, Garcia JV, von Suhr N, Lynch CM, Wilson C, Eiden MV. Construction and properties of retrovirus packaging cells based on gibbon ape leukemia virus. J Virol 1991;65:2220—4.

[21] Swift S, Lorens J, Achacoso P, Nolan GP. Rapid production of retroviruses for efficient gene delivery to mammalian cells using 293T cell-based systems. Curr Protoc Immunol 2001. Chapter 10:Unit 10 7C.

[22] Cavazzana-Calvo M, Hacein-Bey S, de Saint Basile G, Gross F, Yvon E, Nusbaum P, et al. Gene therapy of human severe combined immunodeficiency (SCID)-X1 disease. Science 2000;288:669—72.

[23] Guo X, Wu Y, Hartley RS. MicroRNA-125a represses cell growth by targeting HuR in breast cancer. RNA Biol 2009;6:575—83.

[24] Hacein-Bey-Abina S, Le Deist F, Carlier F, Bouneaud C, Hue C, De Villartay JP, et al. Sustained correction of X-linked severe combined immunodeficiency by ex vivo gene therapy. N Engl J Med 2002;346:1185—93.

[25] Administration UFaD. Cellular & gene therapy guidances. July 18, 2014. https://www-fda-govezproxylibrarytuftsedu/BiologicsBloodVaccines/GuidanceComplianceRegulatoryInformation/Guidances/CellularandGeneTherapy/.

[26] Gross G, Gorochov G, Waks T, Eshhar Z. Generation of effector T cells expressing chimeric T cell receptor with antibody type-specificity. Transplant Proc 1989;21:127—30.

[27] Hacein-Bey-Abina S, Pai SY, Gaspar HB, Armant M, Berry CC, Blanche S, et al. A modified gamma-retrovirus vector for X-linked severe combined immunodeficiency. N Engl J Med 2014;371:1407—17.

[28] Steffens CM, Hope TJ. Recent advances in the understanding of HIV accessory protein function. AIDS 2001;15(Suppl. 5):S21—6.

[29] Wei P, Garber ME, Fang SM, Fischer WH, Jones KA. A novel CDK9-associated C-type cyclin interacts directly with HIV-1 Tat and mediates its high-affinity, loop-specific binding to TAR RNA. Cell 1998;92:451—62.

[30] Rucker E, Grivel JC, Munch J, Kirchhoff F, Margolis L. Vpr and Vpu are important for efficient human immunodeficiency virus type 1 replication and CD4+ T-cell depletion in human lymphoid tissue ex vivo. J Virol 2004;78:12689—93.

[31] Zufferey R, Nagy D, Mandel RJ, Naldini L, Trono D. Multiply attenuated lentiviral vector achieves efficient gene delivery in vivo. Nat Biotechnol 1997;15:871—5.

[32] Zufferey R, Dull T, Mandel RJ, Bukovsky A, Quiroz D, Naldini L, et al. Self-inactivating lentivirus vector for safe and efficient in vivo gene delivery. J Virol 1998;72:9873—80.

[33] Naldini L, Blomer U, Gage FH, Trono D, Verma IM. Efficient transfer, integration, and sustained long-term expression of the transgene in adult rat brains injected with a lentiviral vector. Proc Natl Acad Sci USA 1996;93:11382—8.

[34] Miyoshi H, Takahashi M, Gage FH, Verma IM. Stable and efficient gene transfer into the retina using an HIV-based lentiviral vector. Proc Natl Acad Sci USA 1997;94:10319—23.

[35] Kafri T, Blomer U, Peterson DA, Gage FH, Verma IM. Sustained expression of genes delivered directly into liver and muscle by lentiviral vectors. Nat Genet 1997;17:314—7.

[36] Vannucci L, Lai M, Chiuppesi F, Ceccherini-Nelli L, Pistello M. Viral vectors: a look back and ahead on gene transfer technology. New Microbiol 2013;36:1–22.

[37] Varmus HE, Quintrell N, Ortiz S. Retroviruses as mutagens: insertion and excision of a nontransforming provirus alter expression of a resident transforming provirus. Cell 1981;25:23–36.

[38] Howe SJ, Mansour MR, Schwarzwaelder K, Bartholomae C, Hubank M, Kempski H, et al. Insertional mutagenesis combined with acquired somatic mutations causes leukemogenesis following gene therapy of SCID-X1 patients. J Clin Invest 2008;118:3143–50.

[39] Hacein-Bey-Abina S, Garrigue A, Wang GP, Soulier J, Lim A, Morillon E, et al. Insertional oncogenesis in 4 patients after retrovirus-mediated gene therapy of SCID-X1. J Clin Invest 2008;118:3132–42.

[40] Stein S, Ott MG, Schultze-Strasser S, Jauch A, Burwinkel B, Kinner A, et al. Genomic instability and myelodysplasia with monosomy 7 consequent to EVI1 activation after gene therapy for chronic granulomatous disease. Nat Med 2010;16:198–204.

[41] Bonifant CL, Jackson HJ, Brentjens RJ, Curran KJ. Toxicity and management in CAR T-cell therapy. Mol Ther Oncolytics 2016;3:16011.

[42] Grandgenett DP, Vora AC. Site-specific nicking at the avian retrovirus LTR circle junction by the viral pp32 DNA endonuclease. Nucleic Acids Res 1985;13:6205–21.

[43] Hoboken N. HIV-1 integrase: mechanism and inhibitor design. Wiley; 2011.

[44] Kelly PF, Carrington J, Nathwani A, Vanin EF. RD114-pseudotyped oncoretroviral vectors. Biological and physical properties. Ann N Y Acad Sci 2001;938:262–76. discussion 76-7.

[45] Mulligan RC. The basic science of gene therapy. Science 1993;260:926–32.

[46] Cosset FL, Takeuchi Y, Battini JL, Weiss RA, Collins MK. High-titer packaging cells producing recombinant retroviruses resistant to human serum. J Virol 1995;69:7430–6.

[47] Mann R, Mulligan RC, Baltimore D. Construction of a retrovirus packaging mutant and its use to produce helper-free defective retrovirus. Cell 1983;33:153–9.

[48] Watanabe S, Temin HM. Construction of a helper cell line for avian reticuloendotheliosis virus cloning vectors. Mol Cell Biol 1983;3:2241–9.

[49] Danos O. Construction of retroviral packaging cell lines. In: Collins M, editor. Methods in molecular biology, vol. 8. Clifton, NJ: The Humana Press Inc; 1991. p. 17–26.

[50] Coffin JM, Hughes SH, Varmus HE. The interactions of retroviruses and their hosts. In: Coffin JM, Hughes SH, Varmus HE, editors. Retroviruses. NY: Cold Spring Harbor; 1997.

[51] Andrake MD, Skalka AM. Retroviral integrase: then and now. Annu Rev Virol 2015;2:241–64.

[52] Cullen BR, Lomedico PT, Ju G. Transcriptional interference in avian retroviruses–implications for the promoter insertion model of leukaemogenesis. Nature 1984;307:241–5.

[53] Iwakuma T, Cui Y, Chang LJ. Self-inactivating lentiviral vectors with U3 and U5 modifications. Virology 1999;261:120–32.

[54] Zhou H, Rainey GJ, Wong SK, Coffin JM. Substrate sequence selection by retroviral integrase. J Virol 2001;75:1359–70.

[55] Apolonia L, Waddington SN, Fernandes C, Ward NJ, Bouma G, Blundell MP, et al. Stable gene transfer to muscle using non-integrating lentiviral vectors. Mol Ther 2007;15:1947–54.

[56] Farnet CM, Haseltine WA. Circularization of human immunodeficiency virus type 1 DNA in vitro. J Virol 1991;65:6942–52.

[57] Butler SL, Hansen MS, Bushman FD. A quantitative assay for HIV DNA integration in vivo. Nat Med 2001;7:631–4.

[58] Verghese SC, Goloviznina NA, Skinner AM, Lipps HJ, Kurre PS. MAR sequence confers long-term mitotic stability on non-integrating lentiviral vector episomes without selection. Nucleic Acids Res 2014;42:e53.

[59] Jin C, Fotaki G, Ramachandran M, Nilsson B, Essand M, Yu D. Safe engineering of CAR T cells for adoptive cell therapy of cancer using long-term episomal gene transfer. EMBO Mol Med 2016;8:702–11.

[60] Singh H, Huls H, Kebriaei P, Cooper LJ. A new approach to gene therapy using Sleeping Beauty to genetically modify clinical-grade T cells to target CD19. Immunol Rev 2014;257:181–90.

[61] Singh H, Figliola MJ, Dawson MJ, Olivares S, Zhang L, Yang G, et al. Manufacture of clinical-grade CD19-specific T cells stably expressing chimeric antigen receptor using Sleeping Beauty system and artificial antigen presenting cells. PLoS One 2013;8:e64138.

[62] Nakazawa Y, Matsuda K, Kurata T, Sueki A, Tanaka M, Sakashita K, et al. Anti-proliferative effects of T cells expressing a ligand-based chimeric antigen receptor against CD116 on CD34(+) cells of juvenile myelomonocytic leukemia. J Hematol Oncol 2016;9:27.

[63] Kebriaei P, Izsvak Z, Narayanavari SA, Singh H, Ivics Z. Gene therapy with the sleeping beauty transposon system. Trends Genet 2017;33:852–70.

[64] Davidson AE, Gratsch TE, Morell MH, O'Shea KS, Krull CE. Use of the Sleeping Beauty transposon system for stable gene expression in mouse embryonic stem cells. Cold Spring Harb Protoc 2009;2009. pdb prot5270.

[65] Kalos M, Levine BL, Porter DL, Katz S, Grupp SA, Bagg A, et al. T cells with chimeric antigen receptors have potent antitumor effects and can establish memory in patients with advanced leukemia. Sci Transl Med 2011;3.95ra73.

[66] Porter DL, Levine BL, Kalos M, Bagg A, June CH. Chimeric antigen receptor-modified T cells in chronic lymphoid leukemia. N Engl J Med 2011;365:725–33.

[67] Milone MC, Fish JD, Carpenito C, Carroll RG, Binder GK, Teachey D, et al. Chimeric receptors

containing CD137 signal transduction domains mediate enhanced survival of T cells and increased antileukemic efficacy in vivo. Mol Ther 2009;17:1453—64.

[68] Carpenito C, Milone MC, Hassan R, Simonet JC, Lakhal M, Suhoski MM, et al. Control of large, established tumor xenografts with genetically retargeted human T cells containing CD28 and CD137 domains. Proc Natl Acad Sci USA 2009;106:3360—5.

[69] Zhang C, Wang Z, Yang Z, Wang M, Li S, Li Y, et al. Phase I escalating-dose trial of CAR-T therapy targeting CEA(+) metastatic colorectal cancers. Mol Ther 2017; 25:1248—58.

[70] Kochenderfer JN, Feldman SA, Zhao Y, Xu H, Black MA, Morgan RA, et al. Construction and preclinical evaluation of an anti-CD19 chimeric antigen receptor. J Immunother 2009;32:689—702.

[71] Lee DW, Kochenderfer JN, Stetler-Stevenson M, Cui YK, Delbrook C, Feldman SA, et al. T cells expressing CD19 chimeric antigen receptors for acute lymphoblastic leukaemia in children and young adults: a phase 1 dose-escalation trial. Lancet 2015;385:517—28.

[72] Pizzitola I, Anjos-Afonso F, Rouault-Pierre K, Lassailly F, Tettamanti S, Spinelli O, et al. Chimeric antigen receptors against CD33/CD123 antigens efficiently target primary acute myeloid leukemia cells in vivo. Leukemia 2014;28:1596—605.

[73] Wilkie S, Picco G, Foster J, Davies DM, Julien S, Cooper L, et al. Retargeting of human T cells to tumor-associated MUC1: the evolution of a chimeric antigen receptor. J Immunol 2008;180:4901—9.

[74] Ahmed N, Ratnayake M, Savoldo B, Perlaky L, Dotti G, Wels WS, et al. Regression of experimental medulloblastoma following transfer of HER2-specific T cells. Cancer Res 2007;67:5957—64.

[75] Ahmed N, Brawley VS, Hegde M, Robertson C, Ghazi A, Gerken C, et al. Human epidermal growth factor receptor 2 (HER2) -specific chimeric antigen receptor-modified T cells for the immunotherapy of HER2-positive sarcoma. J Clin Oncol 2015;33:1688—96.

[76] Maher J, Brentjens RJ, Gunset G, Riviere I, Sadelain M. Human T-lymphocyte cytotoxicity and proliferation directed by a single chimeric TCRzeta/CD28 receptor. Nat Biotechnol 2002;20:70—5.

[77] Israeli RS, Powell CT, Corr JG, Fair WR, Heston WD. Expression of the prostate-specific membrane antigen. Cancer Res 1994;54:1807—11.

[78] Weijtens ME, Willemsen RA, Valerio D, Stam K, Bolhuis RL. Single chain Ig/gamma gene-redirected human T lymphocytes produce cytokines, specifically lyse tumor cells, and recycle lytic capacity. J Immunol 1996;157:836—43.

[79] Katz SC, Burga RA, McCormack E, Wang LJ, Mooring W, Point GR, et al. Phase I hepatic immunotherapy for metastases study of intra-arterial chimeric antigen receptor-modified T-cell therapy for CEA$^+$ liver metastases. Clin Cancer Res 2015;21:3149—59.

[80] Riviere I, Brose K, Mulligan RC. Effects of retroviral vector design on expression of human adenosine deaminase in murine bone marrow transplant recipients engrafted with genetically modified cells. Proc Natl Acad Sci USA 1995;92:6733—7.

[81] Sadelain M, Wang CH, Antoniou M, Grosveld F, Mulligan RC. Generation of a high-titer retroviral vector capable of expressing high levels of the human beta-globin gene. Proc Natl Acad Sci USA 1995;92: 6728—32.

[82] Hurford Jr RK, Dranoff G, Mulligan RC, Tepper RI. Gene therapy of metastatic cancer by in vivo retroviral gene targeting. Nat Genet 1995;10:430—5.

[83] Parker LL, Do MT, Westwood JA, Wunderlich JR, Dudley ME, Rosenberg SA, et al. Expansion and characterization of T cells transduced with a chimeric receptor against ovarian cancer. Hum Gene Ther 2000;11: 2377—87.

[84] Kershaw MH, Westwood JA, Parker LL, Wang G, Eshhar Z, Mavroukakis SA, et al. A phase I study on adoptive immunotherapy using gene-modified T cells for ovarian cancer. Clin Cancer Res 2006;12:6106—15.

[85] Hwu P, Shafer GE, Treisman J, Schindler DG, Gross G, Cowherd R, et al. Lysis of ovarian cancer cells by human lymphocytes redirected with a chimeric gene composed of an antibody variable region and the Fc receptor gamma chain. J Exp Med 1993;178:361—6.

[86] Hwu P, Yang JC, Cowherd R, Treisman J, Shafer GE, Eshhar Z, et al. In vivo antitumor activity of T cells redirected with chimeric antibody/T-cell receptor genes. Cancer Res 1995;55:3369—73.

[87] McGuinness RP, Ge Y, Patel SD, Kashmiri SV, Lee HS, Hand PH, et al. Anti-tumor activity of human T cells expressing the CC49-zeta chimeric immune receptor. Hum Gene Ther 1999;10:165—73.

[88] Hege KM, Bergsland EK, Fisher GA, Nemunaitis JJ, Warren RS, McArthur JG, et al. Safety, tumor trafficking and immunogenicity of chimeric antigen receptor (CAR)-T cells specific for TAG-72 in colorectal cancer. J Immunother Cancer 2017;5:22.

[89] Guest RD, Kirillova N, Mowbray S, Gornall H, Rothwell DG, Cheadle EJ, et al. Definition and application of good manufacturing process-compliant production of CEA-specific chimeric antigen receptor expressing T-cells for phase I/II clinical trial. Cancer Immunol Immunother 2014;63:133—45.

[90] Chmielewski M, Abken H. CAR T cells releasing IL-18 convert to T-bet(high) FoxO1(low) effectors that exhibit augmented activity against advanced solid tumors. Cell Rep 2017;21:3205—19.

[91] Kershaw MH, Westwood JA, Darcy PK. Gene-engineered T cells for cancer therapy. Nat Rev Cancer 2013;13:525—41.

[92] Dotti G, Gottschalk S, Savoldo B, Brenner MK. Design and development of therapies using chimeric antigen receptor-expressing T cells. Immunol Rev 2014;257: 107—26.

[93] Gross G, Waks T, Eshhar Z. Expression of immunoglobulin-T-cell receptor chimeric molecules as functional receptors with antibody-type specificity. Proc Natl Acad Sci USA 1989;86:10024—8.

[94] Sadelain M, Brentjens R, Riviere I. The basic principles of chimeric antigen receptor design. Cancer Discov 2013;3: 388—98.

[95] Brentjens RJ, Riviere I, Park JH, Davila ML, Wang X, Stefanski J, et al. Safety and persistence of adoptively transferred autologous CD19-targeted T cells in patients with relapsed or chemotherapy refractory B-cell leukemias. Blood 2011;118:4817—28.

[96] Emtage PC, Lo AS, Gomes EM, Liu DL, Gonzalo-Daganzo RM, Junghans RP. Second-generation anti-carcinoembryonic antigen designer T cells resist activation-induced cell death, proliferate on tumor contact, secrete cytokines, and exhibit superior antitumor activity in vivo: a preclinical evaluation. Clin Cancer Res 2008;14:8112—22.

[97] Zhong XS, Matsushita M, Plotkin J, Riviere I, Sadelain M. Chimeric antigen receptors combining 4-1BB and CD28 signaling domains augment PI3kinase/AKT/Bcl-XL activation and CD8$^+$ T cell-mediated tumor eradication. Mol Ther 2010;18:413—20.

[98] Smith C, Okern G, Rehan S, Beagley L, Lee SK, Aarvak T, et al. Ex vivo expansion of human T cells for adoptive immunotherapy using the novel Xeno-free CTS Immune Cell Serum Replacement. Clin Transl Immunology 2015;4:e31.

[99] Almasbak H, Aarvak T, Vemuri MC. CAR T cell therapy: a game changer in cancer treatment. J Immunol Res 2016; 2016:5474602.

[100] Barrett DM, Singh N, Liu X, Jiang S, June CH, Grupp SA, et al. Relation of clinical culture method to T-cell memory status and efficacy in xenograft models of adoptive immunotherapy. Cytotherapy 2014;16:619—30.

[101] Zhao Y, Wang QJ, Yang S, Kochenderfer JN, Zheng Z, Zhong X, et al. A herceptin-based chimeric antigen receptor with modified signaling domains leads to enhanced survival of transduced T lymphocytes and antitumor activity. J Immunol 2009;183: 5563—74.

[102] Moritz D, Wels W, Mattern J, Groner B. Cytotoxic T lymphocytes with a grafted recognition specificity for ERBB2-expressing tumor cells. Proc Natl Acad Sci USA 1994;91:4318—22.

[103] Stancovski I, Schindler DG, Waks T, Yarden Y, Sela M, Eshhar Z. Targeting of T lymphocytes to Neu/HER2-expressing cells using chimeric single chain Fv receptors. J Immunol 1993;151:6577—82.

[104] Till BG, Jensen MC, Wang J, Qian X, Gopal AK, Maloney DG, et al. CD20-specific adoptive immunotherapy for lymphoma using a chimeric antigen receptor with both CD28 and 4-1BB domains: pilot clinical trial results. Blood 2012;119:3940—50.

[105] Li Y, Kurlander RJ. Comparison of anti-CD3 and anti-CD28-coated beads with soluble anti-CD3 for expanding human T cells: differing impact on CD8 T cell phenotype and responsiveness to restimulation. J Transl Med 2010;8:104.

[106] Dalal AR, Homsy S, Balkhi MY. Third-generation human epidermal growth factor receptor 2 chimeric antigen receptor expression on human T cells improves with two-signal activation. Hum Gene Ther 2018.

[107] Wang A, Pan D, Lee YH, Martinez GJ, Feng XH, Dong C. Cutting edge: smad2 and Smad4 regulate TGF-beta-mediated Il9 gene expression via EZH2 displacement. J Immunol 2013;191:4908—12.

[108] Matz MV, Fradkov AF, Labas YA, Savitsky AP, Zaraisky AG, Markelov ML, et al. Fluorescent proteins from nonbioluminescent Anthozoa species. Nat Biotechnol 1999;17:969—73.

[109] Shaner NC, Campbell RE, Steinbach PA, Giepmans BN, Palmer AE, Tsien RY. Improved monomeric red, orange and yellow fluorescent proteins derived from Discosoma sp. red fluorescent protein. Nat Biotechnol 2004; 22:1567—72.

[110] Morozova KS, Piatkevich KD, Gould TJ, Zhang J, Bewersdorf J, Verkhusha VV. Far-red fluorescent protein excitable with red lasers for flow cytometry and superresolution STED nanoscopy. Biophys J 2010;99:L13—5.

[111] Piatkevich KD, Verkhusha VV. Guide to red fluorescent proteins and biosensors for flow cytometry. Methods Cell Biol 2011;102:431—61.

[112] Niles RM, Wilhelm SA, Steele Jr GD, Burke B, Christensen T, Dexter D, et al. Isolation and characterization of an undifferentiated human colon carcinoma cell line (MIP-101). Cancer Invest 1987;5:545—52.

[113] Dai X, Cheng H, Bai Z, Li J. Breast cancer cell line classification and its relevance with breast tumor subtyping. J Cancer 2017;8:3131—41.

[114] Brunner KT, Mauel J, Cerottini JC, Chapuis B. Quantitative assay of the lytic action of immune lymphoid cells on 51-Cr-labelled allogeneic target cells in vitro; inhibition by isoantibody and by drugs. Immunology 1968; 14:181—96.

[115] Baumgaertner P, Speiser DE, Romero P, Rufer N, Hebeisen M. Chromium-51 (51Cr) release assay to assess human T cells for functional avidity and tumor cell recognition. Bio-protocol 2016;6:1906.

[116] Fu X, Tao L, Rivera A, Williamson S, Song XT, Ahmed N, et al. A simple and sensitive method for measuring tumor-specific T cell cytotoxicity. PLoS One 2010;5: e11867.

[117] Scholler J, Brady TL, Binder-Scholl G, Hwang WT, Plesa G, Hege KM, et al. Decade-long safety and function of retroviral-modified chimeric antigen receptor T cells. Sci Transl Med 2012;4:132ra53.

[118] Kowolik CM, Topp MS, Gonzalez S, Pfeiffer T, Olivares S, Gonzalez N, et al. CD28 costimulation provided through a CD19-specific chimeric antigen receptor enhances in vivo persistence and antitumor efficacy of adoptively transferred T cells. Cancer Res 2006;66:10995—1004.

[119] Stephan MT, Ponomarev V, Brentjens RJ, Chang AH, Dobrenkov KV, Heller G, et al. T cell-encoded CD80 and 4-1BBL induce auto- and transcostimulation,

resulting in potent tumor rejection. Nat Med 2007;13:
1440—9.

[120] Savoldo B, Ramos CA, Liu E, Mims MP, Keating MJ,
Carrum G, et al. CD28 costimulation improves expansion and persistence of chimeric antigen receptor-
modified T cells in lymphoma patients. J Clin Invest
2011;121:1822—6.

[121] Lim WA, June CH. The principles of engineering immune cells to treat cancer. Cell 2017;168:724—40.

[122] Shultz LD, Ishikawa F, Greiner DL. Humanized mice in
translational biomedical research. Nat Rev Immunol
2007;7:118—30.

[123] Flanagan SP. 'Nude', a new hairless gene with pleio-
tropic effects in the mouse. Genet Res 1966;8:
295—309.

[124] Li B, Zhang X, Shi S, Zhao L, Zhang D, Qian W, et al.
Construction and characterization of a bispecific
anti-CD20 antibody with potent antitumor activity
against B-cell lymphoma. Cancer Res 2010;70:
6293—302.

[125] Shultz LD, Schweitzer PA, Christianson SW, Gott B,
Schweitzer IB, Tennent B, et al. Multiple defects in innate
and adaptive immunologic function in NOD/LtSz-scid
mice. J Immunol 1995;154:180—91.

[126] Banuelos SJ, Shultz LD, Greiner DL, Burzenski LM,
Gott B, Lyons BL, et al. Rejection of human islets and human HLA-A2.1 transgenic mouse islets by alloreactive

human lymphocytes in immunodeficient NOD-scid
and NOD-Rag1(null)Prf1(null) mice. Clin Immunol
2004;112:273—83.

[127] Sugamura K, Asao H, Kondo M, Tanaka N, Ishii N,
Ohbo K, et al. The interleukin-2 receptor gamma chain:
its role in the multiple cytokine receptor complexes and
T cell development in XSCID. Annu Rev Immunol 1996;
14:179—205.

[128] Macchiarini F, Manz MG, Palucka AK, Shultz LD. Humanized mice: are we there yet? J Exp Med 2005;202:
1307—11.

[129] Shultz LD, Lyons BL, Burzenski LM, Gott B, Chen X,
Chaleff S, et al. Human lymphoid and myeloid cell
development in NOD/LtSz-scid IL2R gamma null mice
engrafted with mobilized human hemopoietic stem
cells. J Immunol 2005;174:6477—89.

[130] Ishikawa F, Yasukawa M, Lyons B, Yoshida S,
Miyamoto T, Yoshimoto G, et al. Development of functional human blood and immune systems in NOD/
SCID/IL2 receptor {gamma} chain(null) mice. Blood
2005;106:1565—73.

[131] Norelli M, Camisa B, Barbiera G, Falcone L, Purevdorj A,
Genua M, et al. Monocyte-derived IL-1 and IL-6 are
differentially required for cytokine-release syndrome
and neurotoxicity due to CAR T cells. Nat Med 2018;
24:739—48.

CHAPTER 4

Production of CAR-T Cells for Clinical Applications

CLINICAL PRODUCTION OF CAR-T CELLS USING GOOD MANUFACTURING PRACTICES

The chimeric antigen receptor (CAR) T-cell therapy requires ex vivo modification of patient-derived T cells with tumor antigen-specific "chimeric antigen receptors" and subsequent transfer of CAR-modified T cells back to the patient (i.e., autologous T-cell transfer). The important steps in CAR therapy, therefore, involves ex vivo expansion, activation, and modification of patient-derived T cells. The modification of T cells require handling retroviral vector stocks (VS) and vector producer cells (VPCs). The entire process is, therefore, performed in good manufacturing practices (GMP) regulated facility following the good manufacturing practices and good clinical laboratory practices with rigorously established standard operating procedures (SOP)/clinical and laboratory protocols especially involving retroviral infections. The facility designated to process T cells for CAR modification must follow the FDA-approved guidelines for good clinical practices, state government regulations, and institutional research policies and procedures. As Fig. 4.1 illustrates, the SOPs are applicable to all steps including patient recruitment, establishing treatment eligibility criteria, leukapheresis, blood processing and T-cell ex vivo expansion, retroviral supernatant freeze/thaw and subsequent infection of primary T cells, laboratory analyses, for example, determining cell viability and percent CAR T-cell modifications, and reinfusion of CAR-T products to the patients. Furthermore, CAR infusion requires follow-up and monitoring of induced CAR T-cell responses in patients, which is performed in accordance with minimal information about T-cell assays (MIATA) guidelines [1] www.miataproject.org. The key points related to MIATA guidelines applicable for CAR therapy include the following:

1. Reporting about the samples, donors, and patients including the techniques used to acquire patient samples, sample processing information, freeze thaw procedures for apheresis, leukapheresis, vector products, material transport, and storage.
2. Reporting about the techniques, assays, materials, reagents, and equipment used for CAR-T production and analyses.
3. Reporting about the data acquisition techniques such as the information about software used in the data acquisition and their setup.
4. Reporting about the biological significance of the results obtained and how that results correlated with the specific disease and CAR T-cell treatment.
5. Reporting about the use of standard operating procedures, compliance with good manufacturing practices, the status and qualifications and level of training of the personnel handling patient samples, retroviral VS and VPCs.
6. Reporting about the adverse outcomes and unexpected results.

PATIENT RECRUITMENT AND ELIGIBILITY CRITERIA FOR RECEIVING CAR T-CELL THERAPY

The first step in CAR-T therapy is the recruitment of patients according to defined set of clinical eligibility criteria. The patient eligibility criteria may differ between cancer types. Therefore, we will demonstrate the patient eligibility for receiving CAR-T treatment by citing examples from the published clinical eligibility criteria adopted in CAR T-cell therapy clinical trials for the patients with B-cell malignancies, ovarian, and metastatic colorectal cancers.

Eligibility Criteria for CD19$^+$ B-Cell Malignancies

The CD19$^+$ B-cell malignancies is heterogenous group of diseases that includes non-Hodgkin's lymphoma (NHL), B-acute lymphoblastic leukemia (B-ALL), and chronic lymphocytic leukemia (CLL). Patients including the children who present with incurable treatment refractory or relapsed CD19$^+$ B-cell

Basics of Chimeric Antigen Receptor (CAR) Immunotherapy. https://doi.org/10.1016/B978-0-12-819573-4.00004-1

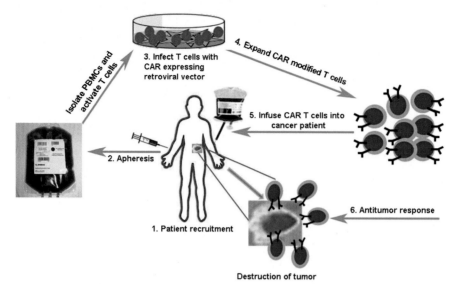

FIG. 4.1 The steps involved in clinical application of CARs. The process of applying CAR therapy begins with the recruitment of patients battling stage IV cancers **(step 1)**. In the next step, patients undergo apheresis. The PBMCs are isolated from the apheresis products. The PBMCs are expanded and activated in ex vivo cultures till a desired T cell number is reached **(step 2)**. T cells are infected with precollected CAR-retroviral particles to modify T-cell receptors. CAR-modified T cells are expanded ex vivo and percent modifications are determined followed by preparing stocks for autologous infusions **(step 3)**. In the final steps, CAR-T cells are reinfused into the patients. The patient is monitored for antitumor response and any potential adverse outcome **(step 4-6)**.

malignancies are eligible to receive CD19-CAR T-cell treatment [2–5]. The patients must have optimal liver and kidney functions. The patient T cells must show optimal functions. Therefore, patient T-cell aliquots are assessed for in vitro expansion. Patient T-cells are expected to demonstrate more than fivefold expansion with CD3/CD28 beads in vitro and above 20% transduction efficiency with CAR lentiviral vectors. However, there are no minimum universally accepted set values for both the expansion and percent modifications of T cells to determine the patient eligibility to receive CAR therapy. The fivefold expansion seems reasonable as expansion properties of T cells determine their potential for activation, the retroviral infection rates, integration of transgene, and the percent modification. The percent modification of CAR-T cells is crucial for the antitumor responses and potentially for generating memory responses. There are no set established clinical guidelines for the required minimum percentage modification of CAR-T cells before a protocol can be approved to conduct clinical trials. However, a minimum range of 5%–20% CAR T-cell modifications seems reasonable especially in case of B-cell malignancies, as favorable results have been achieved even

with lower percentage of CD19-CAR-modified T cells [3].

The patients with CD19$^+$ B-cell malignancies eligible to receive CAR-T therapy must be ineligible to receive autologous and allogeneic stem-cell transplants. However, in B-ALL or NHL CAR trials in which patients who had previously received allogeneic hematopoietic stem-cell transplant were considered eligible post 100 days of transplant [4]. All patients, however, must not present evidences of graft versus host disease and must not require immunosuppression at the time of enrollment. Women who are pregnant or lactating are ineligible to receive CAR therapy. Similarly, patients with active viral infections such as HIV, HCV, and HBV have also been excluded [2–4].

In all patients eligible to receive CAR-T therapy, the serum creatinine levels must be greater or equal to 1.6–2.5 mg/dL, bilirubin greater than 2.0 mg/dL, hemoglobin greater than 9.0 g/dL. WBC and plateletcount must be in the range of 3000/mm^3 and 100,000/mm^3, respectively. Another patient eligibility criterion that has been adopted in CAR-T trials involves eliciting delayed type hypersensitivity cellular immune response to intradermal inoculation of *Candida albicans*, mumps, or tetanus toxoid antigens [6]. The test allows evaluating T-cell response in patents before CAR infusions.

Eligibility Criteria for CAR-T Therapy in Patients With Solid Cancers, e.g., TAG72$^+$ Metastatic Colorectal Cancer, and FR$^+$ Ovarian Cancer

Patient eligibility criteria vary with each cancer type. A common eligibility criterion adopted to date for colorectal and ovarian cancer patients to undergo CAR-T therapy include failure of available standard therapies. The cancer patients must show in their biopsy staining tests the evidences of residual, recurrent, or resected recurrent tumor antigen marker positivity. For example, the ovarian cancer patients' biopsies must show positive staining for the foliate receptor (FR+) [6]. Similarly, in colorectal cancer patients, the TAG72 expression must be detected in 5% of tumor cells and its serum level must be greater than 500 U/mL [7]. In addition, patients must present with metastatic colorectal cancer with at least one liver metastasis. The transaminase levels must be five times the upper limit to normal.

Overall, the serum creatinine levels must be greater or equal to 1.6 mg/dL, bilirubin greater than 2.0 mg/dL, and hemoglobin greater than 9.0 g/dL. The WBC and platelet count must be in the range of 3000/mm^3 and 100,000/mm^3, respectively. In addition, patients must elicit delayed-type hypersensitivity cellular immune response to intradermal inoculation of *Candida albicans*, mumps, or tetanus toxoid antigens [6].

LEUKAPHERESIS AND PATIENT T-CELL ISOLATION

After patients register themselves to receive autologous CAR T-cell therapy, the steps that follow are almost identical across all B-cell malignancies and solid cancers. The procedures are performed in a facility that operates under GMP regulations as discussed in CLINICAL PRODUCTION OF CAR-T CELLSUSING GOOD MANUFACTURINGPRACTICES section. The steps involved in the CAR therapy are depicted in Fig. 4.1.

The Leukapheresis

The amount of blood drawn from the patient depends upon the blood cell count. From patients who have adequate number of WBC count, enough quantity of blood can be drawn for isolating peripheral blood mononuclear cells (PBMCs). A single apheresis product is expected to yield more than a billion WBCs [6]. The peripheral blood can be collected in tubes containing standard anticoagulants (K2EDTA) or in vacutainer tubes (without anticoagulants). The choice depends upon how sooner the sample can be processed. The patient PBMCs are obtained either through Ficoll—Hypaque gradient centrifugation using Ficoll reagent or using automated cell separators (e.g., Cobe Spectra or Fenwal CS-3000) [7—10]. This is followed by washing, activation, and expansion of PBMCs.

Frozen leukapheresis samples. Apart from the fresh leukapheresis samples, patient-derived apheresis products may be frozen for the future use. In such cases, the freeze and thaw procedures are carefully controlled, and SOPs are strictly followed.

Freezing procedure. The apheresis products are washed using an automated cell washer, for example, Cytomate cell washer (Baxter) to deplete red blood cells and platelets. This is followed by their suspension in freezing media and storage in liquid nitrogen.

Thawing procedure. The frozen apheresis products are thawed slowly and washed in PBS using automated washer. The samples are filtered to remove dead cell debris. The PBMCs are suspended in standard cell growth media and activated with CD3/CD28 beads or with anti-OKT3 antibody [11,12].

Activation and Expansion of PBMCs

CD3/CD28 beads method: Patient-derived PBMCs are usually plated at the concentration of 2×10^6/mL in a standard cell growth medium [e.g., AIM-V or XVIVO-15 media supplemented with heat inactivated human serum and IL2 (100—300 IU/mL)] and subjected to activation with CD3/CD28 beads (Dynabeads CD3/CD28 CTS, Thermo Fisher) used in 3:1 bead-to-cell ratio [13—15]. Apart from Invitrogen, the Miltenyi also manufactures MACS GMP TransAct CD3/CD28 beads that can be similarly used to expand and activate patient T cells. The CD3/CD28 bead-mediated activation of T cells in AIM-V media is performed usually for 3 days in the presence of IL2 (100—300 IU/mL) [3,15,16]. In OKT3-mediated T-cell activation, much higher IL2 concentration has been used. In some clinical studies, enriched T cells have been activated with GMP grade anti-CD3 and anti-CD28 beads for only 24 hours [15,17,18]. Yet, in some phase I clinical studies involving B-cell malignancies, the frozen apheresis products after thaw and washing in PBS and filtration step, the cells were incubated with CD3/CD28 beads (Dynabeads CD3/CD28 CTS) at 3:1 ratio for 1—2 hours to enrich CD3$^+$ T cells. In some other studies, CD3$^+$ T-cell enrichment was performed in special bags termed PermaLife bags (OriGen Biomedical) [14]. During the enrichment step, CD3$^+$ T cells bind to the beads. The bead-bound CD3$^+$ T cells were isolated using the magnetic platform, following which cells were suspended in cell culture media [AIM-V or XVIVO-15 media supplemented with serum and IL2 (100 IU/mL)] and incubated at 37°C incubator for 3 days [11,14,17]. The procedure is usually carried out in culture flasks; however, in some studies special PermaLife bags (Ori-Gen Biomedical) have also been used [14].

OKT3: OKT3 has also been used to activate T cells. Ortho Biotech manufactured anti-OKT3 monoclonal antibody has been frequently used at (30−60 µg/mL) concentration to expand patient PBMCs in CAR clinical trials [10]. The OKT3-mediated activation of PBMCs is performed in standard cell culture media composed of AIM-V (Invitrogen) plus 5% human AB serum (available from Valley Biomedical), L-glutamine (2 mmol/L), antibiotics supplement, and human recombinant IL2 manufactured by Chiron or Prometheus [3,6,10,16]. IL2 has been used in variable quantity ranging from 300 to 3000 IU/mL [6,10]. The activation is usually performed for 48−72 hours using the cell culture flasks. Some studies have preferred to use serum-free AIM-V media as well [7].

GENERATION OF CAR-T CELLS

After T cells are activated and expanded with OKT3 or CD3/CD28 beads. These are subjected to transduction procedures with CAR retroviral vectors. However, before the cells can be subjected to transduction, an aliquot of cells can be stained with pan T-cell markers such as CD3, CD4, and CD8 to determine the overall percentage of T-cell subtypes. A more detailed analysis can also be performed such as determining the Treg population and other smaller T-cell subtypes. In addition, a cytokine expression profile and T-cell exhaustion markers can also be examined. All these pieces of information may prove crucial in evaluating postinfusion antitumor T-cell responses in patients. Obtaining these pieces of data may be useful when a new CAR vector is being tested to target novel tumor antigen.

The retroviral transduction procedures applied across various phase I clinical trials may be marginally different due to the choice of reagents, for example, CD3/CD28 beads versus OKT3, kits and chemical reagents, and the techniques employed to produce, collect and store retroviral stocks. Before T cells can be subjected to transduction protocols, the vector stocks containing CAR expression vectors packaged as retroviral or lentiviral particles with predetermined titer are taken out from −80°C freezer and thawed on ice essentially following the SOPs. The detailed account about the choice of vectors commonly used in clinical trials have already been listed and discussed in Chapter 3, VECTORS USED FOR CAR PRODUCTION section. Here, we will elaborate briefly how CARlentiviral

particles are produced and stored before being utilized to infect primary human T cells in actual clinical trials.

Lentivirus production and storage. HIV1-based lentiviral vectors have become a popular choice in CAR therapy. It is important to note that the process to produce gamma retrovirus-based CARs is different from the production of lentiviral-based CARs. The key differences between these two systems have been explained in Chapter 3. Here, we specifically focus on lentiviral production of CARs for clinical applications. Basically, three separate vectors are transfected into a producer cell line, for example, HEK 293-based cell lines to package CARs as lentiviral particles (Fig. 4.2). Vector 1 contains CAR chimeric gene sequences packaged in third-generation lentiviral-based vectors; vector 2 contains lentiviral structural and reverse transcriptase genes; vector 3 contains envelope gene, for example VSV-G, to alter the viral tropism to enable infection of human T cells. All three plasmids are transfected transiently into HEK 293T producer cells in the 3:2:1 ratio, 48 hours later, the supernatants containing replication incompetent viral particle are produced. These can be centrifuged at 28,000 rpm for 2 hours, filtered, quantitated to determine the titer (infection Units), and stored at −80°C. In addition to HEK 293T cell line, there are 293T-based lentiviral packaging cell lines developed as well among which GPRTG is most notable. The GPRTG cell line expresses HIV *Rev*, *Tat*, and *VSV-G* under Tet-off inducible system and expresses HIV *Gag/Pol* constitutively. Because the percent modification of T cells with CARs (transduction efficiency) crucially depends on the titer and quality of virus production, the vector preparation is usually performed in contract with the companies specialized in vector production and vector safety testing, for example, National Gene Vector Laboratory (NGVL) (https://www.ngvbcc.org/Home.action). Once CAR lentiviral vectors are produced with good titer and pass the safety testing, these can be used to modify patient-derived PBMCs.

Lentiviral Transduction

After T-cell enrichment, activation, and expansion with OKT3 or CD3/CD28 beads as described in previous sections, these are subjected to lentiviral transduction procedures. The number of T cells that may be subjected to transduction procedure depends on the viral titer, a desirable range is >5 transduction Units/cell. The number of T cells transduced in clinical trials have ranged from ~5 × 10^7 to ~10 × 10^8. The concentrated lentiviral particles may be diluted in 1:1 ratio with T-cell complete growth medium before applying the actual transduction procedures. The transduction procedure is performed in retronectin-coated tissue culture well

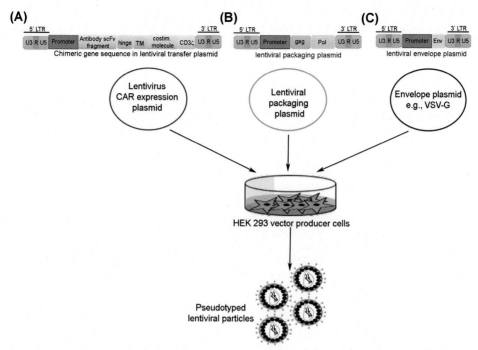

FIG. 4.2 Steps involved in the lentiviral production of CARs. Lentiviral vectors have become popular choice in CAR therapy clinical applications. Three set of vectors are used: lentiviral-based vectors encoding a CAR chimeric gene sequence **(A)**, a lentiviral packaging plasmid **(B)**, and a plasmid encoding envelope gene, for example, VSV-G for pseudotyping lentivirus to infect human T cells **(C)**. These three plasmids are transfected ectopically into clinical grade HEK-293 vector producer cells. The high-titer virus is collected from the producer cells, stored, and submitted for quality control testing including any potential replication-competent virus production. Once the viral supernatants pass the stringent quality control tests, these can be applied to infect patients' T cells.

plates or PermaLife bags. The retronectin solution is prepared in PBS at 1 mg/mL concentration and transferred to plates or bags and incubated overnight at 4°C. Next day, retronectin solution is aspired off following which the plates or bags may be blocked for 30 minutes at room temperature using a blocking solution (2.5% human serum albumin in PBS). This is followed by washings of bags or plates with PBS.

The prior activated patient T cells are combined with lentiviral solution supplemented with IL2 (usually, 300–600 IU/mL) and protamine sulfate (usually, 10 µg/mL), and transferred into retronectin-coated plates or bags.

Lentiviral transduction in CD3/CD28 bead-activated T cells

Before the transduction procedures, patient-derived T cells suspended in flasks or in PermaLife bags can be activated for 24 hours to 3 days with CD3/CD28 beads as discussed in Activation and Expansion of PBMCs

section [3,11,14–18]. The beads are removed using the magnetic platform before subjecting them to lentiviral transduction. However, in a clinical study by Maude et al., the CAR lentiviral vector stocks with predetermined titer was added to enriched T cells before beginning of CD3/CD28 bead-mediated activation, and after 3 days of activation, the viral supernatant was washed and cells in the beads were continued to be expanded in a rocking platform for 8–12 days. At the end of the 8–12-day incubation, beads were removed using a magnetic platform and CAR-T cells were harvested and frozen in fusible media for final release of the product to be reinfused into the patient [3]. Similarly, in a phase I clinical study on CLL conducted at Memorial Sloan-Kettering Cancer Center, Hollyman et al. performed a T-cell enrichment step with CD3/CD28 beads for 1 hour in a rocking platform at room temperature. After T-cell enrichment using a ClinExVivo MPC magnet, the CD3+ T cells were resuspended in a complete growth medium supplemented with IL2 (100 IU/mL) and

CD3/CD28 beads, and transferred into a cell culture incubator. After 3-day incubation, the bead-activated T cells were again enriched using a ClinExVivo MPC magnet, and activated T cells at the concentration of $\sim 2 \times 10^6$ were subjected to first round of lentiviral transduction using retronectin-coated PermaLife bags. The bags were spinoculated for 1 h at 186 g and transferred to 37°C incubator. At day 4, cells were subjected to second round of CAR lentiviral transduction. Subsequently, cells were transferred to larger 2-liter bags for the expansion of transduced T cells using Wave bioreactor. In a WAVE bioreactor fresh media were continuously perfused with increased IL2 concentration from 100 to 500 IU/mL. Finally, when the cell densities reached to $\sim 3 \times 10^7$, cells were debeaded, washed and stored [11]. In a simplified protocol, PBMCs can be activated with CD3/CD28 beads for 24 hours to 3-days. After the activation, cells must be debeaded before subjecting to transduction procedures. Transductions must be performed in retronectin-coated plates using spinoculation method. Basically, $\sim 2 \times 10^6$ T cells can be suspended in lentiviral vector supernatant containing complete media supplemented with IL2, protamine sulfate or polybrene as described in above sections, and spun for 30 minutes at 800 g. Following the completion of spin, cells are returned to 37°C incubator. Usually, 48 hours later cells can be washed and allowed to expand in complete growth media supplemented with IL2 (200 IU/mL) for 10−17 days, at which time point the cell number is expected to reach somewhere in the range of $\sim 2 \times 10^{10}$. It is important that the cell number is counted every 2−3 days and maintained at a concentration of $\sim 1 \times 10^6$ cell/mL and media may be replaced twice weekly before a desirable number of T cells can be achieved. Once the target cell numbers is achieved, CAR-T cells are cryopreserved in infusible media for the autologous infusions.

Retroviral transduction in OKT3-activated T cells

The PBMCs harvested at a density of $\sim 2 \times 10^6$/mL are subjected to OKT3-mediated activation ($\sim 30-60$ μg/mL). The activation is usually carried out for 3 days in flasks in the presence of complete growth media [AIM V or RPMI supplemented with 5% heat-inactivated human serum plus antibiotic cocktail and IL2 (300−3000 IU/mL)] [6,10]. After 3-day activation, cells can be subjected to the transduction procedures. During this time, there is significant expansion of T cells. Before we discuss retroviral transduction procedure, we wanted to briefly summarize how γ-retroviral-based CARs can be produced for clinical applications.

The production of γ-retroviral-based CARs is different from the HIV1-based lentiviral CARs, and the differences have been described in detail in Chapter 3. In several clinical trials, the CAR retroviral vector stocks were generated from PG13 packaging cell line [10,11,19]. To generate a stable clinical grade PG13 CAR VPC, the CAR expression plasmid packaged in γ-retroviral vectors (please refer to the Chapter 3, VECTORS USED FOR CAR PRODUCTION section to learn more about the choice of vectors used in CAR therapy) are transiently transfected into ecotropic cell lines, for example, Phoenix-Eco. The PG13 cells are infected with cell-free retroviral supernatant produced from Phoenix-Eco. Finally, the PG13 CAR vector producer cells are sorted and selected for high viral titer production, and subcloned. The VPC subclone demonstrating higher titer and higher transduction efficiency in infecting human T cells are selected and expanded to make VPC stocks (Fig. 4.3). The PG13 generates GaLV-pseudotyped viral particles capable of infecting human cells [20].

Retroviral transduction of OKT3-activated PBMCs. After day-3 activation, most cells in the culture are T cells. The cells are washed and suspended in diluted CAR retroviral vector stocks as described earlier. The vector stocks are diluted in 1:1 or 1:3 ratio with complete growth media containing IL2 (300−3000 IU/mL) and protamine sulfate (5 μg/mL). Lowering the vector dilution factor has enhanced transduction efficiency possibly due to diluting out of inhibitors in the media. The T cells are suspended in diluted retroviral stocks and seeded at a cell density of $\sim 5 \times 10^7$ to $\sim 10 \times 10^8$ in retronectin (10−20 μg/mL)-coated six well plates [6,10,19]. The choice of cell culture plates depends on the density of cells subjected to retroviral infections. For example, $\sim 1 \times 10^6$ may be seeded in 24 well plates. It is important to note that in some studies instead of protamine sulfate, polybrene (8 μg/mL) has also been used [21]. Furthermore, as described in GENERATION OF CAR-T CELLS section, the clinical grade retroviral batches can be prepared in contract with companies specialized in vector production and safety testing, for example, NGVL. VPCs must be tested for the replication-competent virus (RCR) production, mycoplasma positivity, and integration of proviral vector using qPCR on genomic DNA or southern blot. In addition, all vector stocks are released only after biosafety testing in accordance with FDA guidelines [11].

The T cells seeded in cell culture plates (e.g., six well plates) are sealed and subjected to centrifugation at 1000 g for 1-hour at room temperature as described in Chapter 3, Production of Third-Generation CARlentiviral Particles section, protocol 3. Overall, up to three cycles of

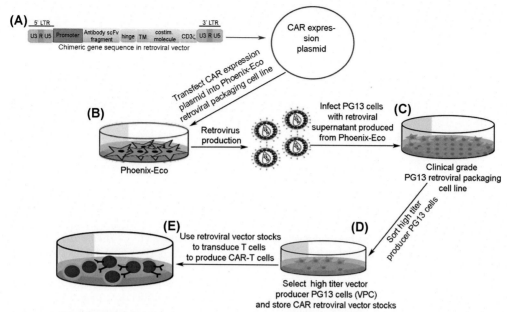

FIG. 4.3 Steps involved in producing a stable clinical grade PG13 CAR vector producer cell line. The CAR chimeric gene sequences are cloned in γ-retroviral-based vectors **(A)**. The CAR vectors can be transiently transfected into ecotropic cell lines, for example, Phoenix-Eco **(B)**. The clinical grade PG13 cell line is infected with cell-free retroviral supernatants produced from Phoenix-Eco **(C)**. The PG13 CAR vector producer cells can be sorted and subcloned for high viral titer production. The VPC subclone demonstrating higher titer production is selected and stored **(D)**. The high-titer retroviral supernatants are used to infect human T cells **(E)**. It is noteworthy that PG13 cell line produces GaLV-pseudotyped viral particles that enable infection of human cells.

transduction can be carried over the course of 24 hours. After the transduction, cells are suspended in complete growth media supplemented with IL2 (300–3000 IU/mL), and placed in 37°C incubator for additional 48–72 hours [10,19]. After 48–72 hours, cells are washed and suspended in complete growth media supplemented with IL2 (100–600 IU/mL) and plated in cell culture flasks or culture bags and transferred back to 37°C incubator, media must be replaced twice a week until a desirable dosage of cell number is achieved usually in 10–14 days [10,19]. In some studies, $CD3^+$ T cells in complete growth media supplemented with IL2 (300–600 IU/mL) were seeded in retronectin-coated bags and suspended in 1:1 dilution with CAR retroviral vector stocks, and placed in 37°C incubator. At day 3, a second round of transduction was performed using freshly prepared retronectin-coated bags; 24 hours later, cells were washed and seeded at $\sim 0.4 \times 10^6$ T-cell density. The cell cultures were maintained at $\sim 0.4 \times 10^6$ T-cell density in complete growth media supplemented with IL2 (100–600 IU/mL) for almost 2 weeks [14,16,21]. Taken together, once the target dose is achieved, CAR-T cells are cryopreserved in infusible media.

INFUSION OF CAR-T CELLS

Once the CAR-modified T-cell products have been prepared, patients are recalled for receiving the CAR infusions. However, before the final products can be released for infusion, certain important requirements associated with the final product release as specified by the FDA guidelines must be met. For example, the cell viability in the final product must be $\sim 70\%$, the CD3 pan T-cell marker must show $\sim 80\%$ positivity, the paramagnetic CD3/CD28 beads must not be in excess of 100 beads per 3×10^6 cells in the final product. However, if the activation is mediated by plate-bound OKT3, no such criterion applies. The RCR production remains a concern that may be produced during CAR T-cell modification or after infusions in patients. The split vector design in which genes encoding the core viral structural and nucleoproteins, envelope proteins, and retroviral reverse transcriptase enzymes are cloned in different plasmids. The split vector design used in CAR-T modifications have greatly minimized the risk of recombination and production of RCR. Similarly, deletion of HIV1 accessory and regulatory genes render RCR nonfunctional in an event recombination does occur. Nevertheless, recent FDA guidelines recommend testing of vector stocks to demonstrate vectors contain less than 1 RCR per patient dose. In addition, the final release product must also be tested for RCR [22,23]. An assay to determine RCR in final release product before infusion can involve detecting VSV-G DNA sequence through PCR or p24 antigen through ELISA [23]. Maude et al. had used VSV-G less than or equal to 50 copies per μg DNA as criteria to determine replication-competent lentivirus [3]. In addition, RCR testing must be performed, an example of which include serological detection of RCR-specific antibodies or PCR-mediated detection of RCR-specific sequences, for example, HIV1-*gag* DNA sequences in patient PBMCs. Moreover, the confirmatory tests on final products must be negative for mycoplasma, bacterial, and fungal contamination. The permitted endotoxin levels in final products must be less than or equal to 3.5 EU/mL. The transduction efficiency must be higher than 20% [2,3,10,19].

Before CAR T-cell infusion, patients with solid cancer such as ovarian or colorectal cancers undergo imaging analysis through computed tomography, magnetic resonance imaging, positron emission tomography, or sonography to examine the tumor burden. After infusion, imaging analysis is again repeated to compare the changes in tumor burden with the CAR-T therapy. In addition, cancer biomarkers such as CA-125 or CEA levels in the serum can also be assesses to evaluate CAR-T dose responses [6,10,16]. After the pretreatment radiological examinations for tumor burden, CAR-T cells are infused to patients. Various amounts of first CAR T-cell doses have been infused to patients with ovarian and colorectal cancers, for example, 3×10^9 per kg, which may be followed by higher doses if dose escalation is required [6]. Similarly, 3×10^8 per kg have used in a separate study followed by higher doses [10].

Patients with $CD19^+$ B-cell malignancies eligible to receive CAR therapy undergo pretreatment with lymphodepleting chemotherapy, for example, fludarabine 25 mg/m^2 for 1−3 days [3−5,24]. This is followed by CAR-T infusion. Patients receive CAR T-cell infusions in multiple cycles. The time between the cycles can vary anywhere between 4 and 6 weeks. For patients with $CD19^+$ B-cell malignancies, CAR T-cell doses have been administered either according to per kg body weight or per m^2. In a trial involving $CD19^+$ ALL, the first dose consisted of 1×10^6 cells that followed an escalating dose of 3×10^6 per kg [4]. Similarly, in a trial involving $CD19^+$ advanced CLL, an initial dose of 1.46×10^5, 1.0×10^7, and 1.6×10^7

per kg were infused in patients that were followed by escalating doses of 1.4×10^7, 5.8×10^8, and 1.1×10^9, respectively [5]. In a separate study, Maude et al. administered CAR T doses composed of 1×10^7 to 10×10^7 per kg [3]. Similarly, in a trial involving anti-CD19 CAR, CAR-T cells were infused per m^2 to patients presented with refractory B-cell NHL. The initial dose consisted of $2 \times 10^7/m^2$, that followed an escalating dose of $1 \times 10^8/m^2$ and $2 \times 10^8/m^2$ [25]. Overall, dose escalations are performed if first dose indicate clinical benefits in terms of tumor cytotoxicity and patient's ability to tolerate higher doses based on toxicity assessments.

For solid cancers, lymphodepleting chemotherapy has also been performed before CAR T-cell infusion. Interestingly, in one study CAR infusion was performed without lymphodepleting chemotherapy [7]. The CAR T-cell numbers (i.e., total T cells including CAR-modified T cells) infused to patients have been either according to per kg body weight or per m^2. For ovarian cancer patients, the initial dose of anti-FR^+ CAR-T cells consisted of 3×10^9 cells, followed by yet higher doses of 1×10^{10} and 3×10^{10}, which is after toxicity assessments revealed no adverse effect [6]. Similarly, in phase I clinical trials in patients with CEA^+ adenocarcinoma, the patients received an initial dose of 1×10^8 second-generation anti-CEA-CAR-T cells. This was followed by higher doses of 1×10^9 and 1×10^{10} [10]. In a phase I/II trial in patients with refractory $HER2^+$ sarcoma, the patients received an initial dose of $1 \times 10^4/m^2$ of second-generation anti-HER2 CAR-T cells, which was followed by higher escalating dose of $1 \times 10^8/m^2$ [16]. Similarly, in a trial involving first-generation anti-TAG72 CAR, patients with $TAG72^+$ colorectal carcinoma with liver metastasis received an initial infusion of 1×10^8 CAR T cells. Followed by dose escalation of 1×10^9 to 1×10^{10} cells [7]. The CAR-T cells in the trial were delivered through hepatic artery catheters.

In majority of clinical trials, CAR T-cell infusions are performed in isolated and sterile rooms. The precautions adopted are in accordance with "immunocompromised subjects." CAR-T cells are generally infused though i.v. drips over 20−30 minutes. Moreover, patients receive various quantitative doses of IL2 regimen though i.v. infusion. However, in some studies, IL2 infusions were avoided [5,25]. Overall, the IL2 doses are given in cycles, and per dose quantity can be between 75,000 and 720,000 IU/kg body weight. However, apart from IL2, IFNα (3 million units) has also been used. IFNα was infused through subcutaneous injections [7]. After the CAR-T infusion, patients are monitored for any adverse events and assessed for antitumor responses.

Patient Monitoring After T-Cell Infusion

After CAR T-cell infusions, patients are monitored for potential adverse outcome as well as clinical benefits according to common terminology criteria for adverse events and response evaluation criteria. The toxicity assessments are usually performed immediately after T-cell infusions, that is, day 0 and can be followed on 1, 2, 4, and 6 weeks. Response evaluation assessments can be followed after 3, 6, 9, and 12 months, and over longer periods of time.

Adverse outcome

Patients receiving CAR-T cells can suffer infusion-related adverse effects. The severities of adverse events are scored from grade 1 to grade 4 using common terminology criteria for adverse events (CTCAE v2.0, v4.0). The adverse events may vary between targeted antigens in cancers. Some of the common side effects observed in patients with CAR T-cell infusions include allergic reactions, chills/nausea, and high-grade fevers [2,5,26]. In addition, patients have been reported to show consistently high lactate dehydrogenase (LDH) levels in serum [26]. LDH is an enzyme that converts pyruvate into lactate during glycolysis under hypoxic conditions of tumors [27]. It is detectable in the serum, and human cancers often present with high LDH levels, which are indicative of tumor burden [28]. Patients may also develop sepsis due to contamination in the CAR-T products. In worst cases, patient may also suffer vital organ failure. Therefore, patients are monitored regularly for toxicity assessments involving routine tests, physical examinations, and organ functions. Therefore, necessary remedial measures are listed in the approved clinical protocols that also list the procedures that are put into place to mitigate the adverse outcomes.

A potentially life-threatening condition experienced in CAR trials is cytokine release syndrome (CRS) that can evolve into macrophage activation syndrome, which is associated with high ferritin levels [26]. The symptoms of CRS are similar to what is observed with excessive immune activation. Patients experiencing CRS are presented with highly elevated levels of inflammatory cytokines such as IFNγ, IL6, IL2, IL1, Ferritin, and C-reactive protein.

Response evaluation in solid cancers

CAR T-mediated response evaluations in solid cancers are determined according to response evaluation criteria in solid tumors (RECIST) [29,30] and immune-modified response evaluation criteria in solid tumors (imRECIST) [31]. RECIST guidelines were originally introduced to score the benefits of chemotherapy and other cancer therapeutics in solid cancers [32,33]. With the recent success of CARs and other immunotherapy drugs especially checkpoint receptor blockade inhibitory drugs, immune-mediated response evaluations adopted several new criteria while retaining some of the already revised RECIST guidelines [31]. One of the most important criteria to evaluate anticancer treatments is assessing changes in tumor burden. The revised RECIST guidelines have inserted following notable criteria assessments: (1) Tumor burden and response to therapy. The number of target lesions to assess treatment response has been set at five in total and two lesions per organ (to serve as representation for all organs involved). (2) Assessment of pathological lymph node involved by the solid tumor. The short axes measurements of lymph node by axial CT scan measuring ≥ 15 mm should be set as baseline to evaluate objective tumor burden regression.

Evaluation of solid tumor burden. Referencing the previously defined parameters as baseline for tumor burden. Anticancer treatment can result in complete remission (CR) or partial response or progressive disease (PD). A patient is set to have entered complete remission if identified tumor lesions completely disappears and pathologic lymph node shrunk to 10 mm size on short axis. If the sum of diameters of identified lesion revealed a shrinkage of 30% of the identified lesions, patient has achieved only partial response. In contrast, if the sum of diameters of identified lesion revealed an increase of 20%, patient is declared to have progressive disease. Besides, an increase of 5 mm in target lesion as well as appearance of new lesions is included to assess PD.

Tumor burden in B-cell malignancies and response evaluations

The amount of tumor burden in B-cell malignancies is usually calculated in bone marrow, blood, and secondary lymphoid organs. The estimate of B cancer cells in bone marrow is based on marrow biopsy and aspirate specimen. The marrow mass conversion into number of cells applies following formula: 1 kg marrow mass $= 10^{12}$ cells. The marrow weight is assigned as 5% of the total body weight in healthy adults [34]. The percentage of B-cell cancers in blood is determined through flow cytometry using surface markers to identify clonal malignant B cells. The response assessment in case of B-cell malignancies may be performed within few days after the CAR-T infusions and in every

3 months for 2 years according to standard care and practices [2]. In one study, response assessment after CD19-CAR infusion in ALL patients was performed 4 days postinfusion [4]. The minimal residual disease negative in case of B-cell malignancies was defined when marrow blast count falls to 0.01% determined by the flow cytometry analysis. In contrast, complete response to CAR-T treatment was defined when marrow blast count is less than 5% and absence of circulating blasts. However, when these set criteria of complete response are not met, patients are defined to have stable disease. The progressive disease was defined when peripheral blood blast count increases to greater than 50% [4]. In case of Hodgkin's and non-Hodgkin's lymphoma, the treatment response is evaluated according to revised response criteria for malignant lymphoma adopted in 2007 [35]. The original response criteria for malignant lymphoma were proposed in 1999 by the international working group composed of clinicians, radiologists, and pathologists [36]. The revised recommendations have been widely adopted. The response evaluations are mostly related to the assessment of overall response rate or complete remission (CR) in clinical trials using imaging techniques especially positron emission tomographic (PET) scanning. PET is strongly recommended for lymphoma patients especially in diffuse large B-cell lymphoma (DLBCL) and Hodgkin's lymphoma before the CAR-T treatment to assess the extent of the disease. It is recommended that PET be performed 6–8 weeks postinfusion [37,38]. A complete absence of physical evidence of symptoms and clinical disease indicate a CR. When the PET scan is confirmed to be negative after treatment, patient is set to have achieved CR despite the residual mass may be detected. The lymph nodes and nodal mass detected in the prior assessment of disease must have regressed to less than 1.5 cm on transverse diameter when analyzed by CT. Bone marrow assessment to evaluate response is recommended for less common lymphoma subtypes such as marginal zone lymphoma and DLBCL, and according to the revised criteria, a histologically normal bone marrow with less than 2% clonal B-cell blasts detected through flow cytometry should be considered normal. Criteria for stable disease in lymphoma: A patient with lymphoma is set to have stable disease if PET scan after CAR treatment appears positive in the previously positive identified areas with no indication of change in size or involvement of new areas posttreatment. Criteria for PD in lymphoma patients after treatment: A patient is set to have progressive disease if new lesions are detected with the size more than 1.5 cm; similarly, after treatment if PET scan reveals uptake of fluorodeoxyglucose (FDG) in new areas; in addition, if lymph node size increases by 50% in previously identified node having a size of more than 1 cm in short axis.

Other techniques used to assess tumor responses to CAR-T therapy

Apart from the imaging techniques such as MRI, CT, or F-FDG PET scans for optical assessment of lesions. The FDG-PET assesses tumor metabolism. Several other important analyses are performed postinfusions to determine (1) the persistence of CAR-T cells in patients, (2) effector cytokine production, and (3) cancer regression. The CAR T-cell persistence in vivo in patients can be assessed by isolating PBMCs aliquots from patients and subjecting them to flow cytometry analysis, immunostaining analysis, or simply a qPCR or qRT-PCR. The results obtained can help conclude if the CAR-T cells have been in recirculation and expanding. The CAR T-cell persistence at tumor sites in case of solid cancers and lymphoma can be determined by resecting tumors and employing qPCR or flow cytometry analysis or immunostaining techniques. That can help evaluating if the CAR-T cells have trafficked to tumor targets. In case of B-cell malignancies, bone marrow can be similarly examined. Moreover, PBMCs or BM infiltrates or resurrected tumors can be analyzed directly for effector cytokine production employing either ELISA or flow cytometry method. Technically, PBMC aliquots from patients or resected tumors can be processed to single-cell suspensions. The CAR-T cells can be surface stained followed by internal staining using fluorophore-conjugated antibodies against specific cytokines. Utilizing gating strategies, cytokine production can be determined and quantitated. The in vivo persistence can also be monitored using advanced imaging techniques such as Vectra Polaris (PerkinElmer) pathology imaging system that can help to quantify, determine T-cell subtypes, visualize, identify, and analyze CAR-T cell in tumor specimen. The in vivo persistence can be monitored for months and years together to help correlating CAR-T persistence with the cancer regression and patient survival. The tumor regression is usually confirmed through radiological examinations.

Taken together, writing a comprehensive clinical protocol forms an essential component of the successful conduct of CAR-T clinical trials in patients. With recent advances in imaging techniques and flow cytometry-based techniques, the real-time monitoring of CAR-T-mediated responses and tumor regressions can be confidently scored and reported.

REFERENCES

[1] Janetzki S, Britten CM, Kalos M, Levitsky HI, Maecker HT, Melief CJ, et al. "MIATA"-minimal information about T cell assays. Immunity 2009;31:527—8.

[2] Porter DL, Levine BL, Kalos M, Bagg A, June CH. Chimeric antigen receptor-modified T cells in chronic lymphoid leukemia. N Engl J Med 2011;365:725—33.

[3] Maude SL, Frey N, Shaw PA, Aplenc R, Barrett DM, Bunin NJ, et al. Chimeric antigen receptor T cells for sustained remissions in leukemia. N Engl J Med 2014;371:1507—17.

[4] Lee DW, Kochenderfer JN, Stetler-Stevenson M, Cui YK, Delbrook C, Feldman SA, et al. T cells expressing CD19 chimeric antigen receptors for acute lymphoblastic leukaemia in children and young adults: a phase 1 dose-escalation trial. Lancet 2015;385:517—28.

[5] Kalos M, Levine BL, Porter DL, Katz S, Grupp SA, Bagg A, et al. T cells with chimeric antigen receptors have potent antitumor effects and can establish memory in patients with advanced leukemia. Sci Transl Med 2011;3:95ra73.

[6] Kershaw MH, Westwood JA, Parker LL, Wang G, Eshhar Z, Mavroukakis SA, et al. A phase I study on adoptive immunotherapy using gene-modified T cells for ovarian cancer. Clin Cancer Res 2006;12:6106—15.

[7] Hege KM, Bergsland EK, Fisher GA, Nemunaitis JJ, Warren RS, McArthur JG, et al. Safety, tumor trafficking and immunogenicity of chimeric antigen receptor (CAR)-T cells specific for TAG-72 in colorectal cancer. J Immunother Cancer 2017;5:22.

[8] Mehta J, Singhal S, Gordon L, Tallman M, Williams S, Luyun R, et al. Cobe Spectra is superior to Fenwal CS 3000 Plus for collection of hematopoietic stem cells. Bone Marrow Transplant 2002;29:563—7.

[9] Perseghin P, Dassi M, Balduzzi A, Rovelli A, Bonanomi S, Uderzo C. Mononuclear cell collection in patients undergoing extra-corporeal photo-chemotherapy for acute and chronic graft-vs.-host-disease (GvHD): comparison between COBE Spectra version 4.7 and 6.0 (AutoPBSC). J Clin Apher 2002;17:65—71.

[10] Katz SC, Burga RA, McCormack E, Wang LJ, Mooring W, Point GR, et al. Phase I hepatic immunotherapy for metastases study of intra-arterial chimeric antigen receptor-modified T-cell therapy for CEA$^+$ liver metastases. Clin Cancer Res 2015;21:3149—59.

[11] Hollyman D, Stefanski J, Przybylowski M, Bartido S, Borquez-Ojeda O, Taylor C, et al. Manufacturing validation of biologically functional T cells targeted to CD19 antigen for autologous adoptive cell therapy. J Immunother 2009;32:169—80.

[12] Tran CA, Burton L, Russom D, Wagner JR, Jensen MC, Forman SJ, et al. Manufacturing of large numbers of patient-specific T cells for adoptive immunotherapy: an approach to improving product safety, composition, and production capacity. J Immunother 2007;30:644—54.

[13] Dalal AR, Homsy S, Balkhi MY. Third-generation human epidermal growth factor receptor 2 chimeric antigen receptor expression on human T cells improves with two-signal activation. Hum Gene Ther 2018;29:845—52.

[14] Tumaini B, Lee DW, Lin T, Castiello L, Stroncek DF, Mackall C, et al. Simplified process for the production of anti-CD19-CAR-engineered T cells. Cytotherapy 2013;15:1406—15.

[15] Milone MC, Fish JD, Carpenito C, Carroll RG, Binder GK, Teachey D, et al. Chimeric receptors containing CD137 signal transduction domains mediate enhanced survival of T cells and increased antileukemic efficacy in vivo. Mol Ther 2009;17:1453—64.

[16] Ahmed N, Brawley VS, Hegde M, Robertson C, Ghazi A, Gerken C, et al. Human epidermal growth factor receptor 2 (HER2) -specific chimeric antigen receptor-modified T cells for the immunotherapy of HER2-positive sarcoma. J Clin Oncol 2015;33:1688—96.

[17] Levine BL, Humeau LM, Boyer J, MacGregor RR, Rebello T, Lu X, et al. Gene transfer in humans using a conditionally replicating lentiviral vector. Proc Natl Acad Sci U S A 2006;103:17372—7.

[18] Levine BL, Mosca JD, Riley JL, Carroll RG, Vahey MT, Jagodzinski LL, et al. Antiviral effect and ex vivo CD4$^+$ T cell proliferation in HIV-positive patients as a result of CD28 costimulation. Science 1996;272:1939—43.

[19] Katz SC, Burga RA, Naheed S, Licata LA, Thorn M, Osgood D, et al. Anti-KIT designer T cells for the treatment of gastrointestinal stromal tumor. J Transl Med 2013;11:46.

[20] Miller AD, Garcia JV, von Suhr N, Lynch CM, Wilson C, Eiden MV. Construction and properties of retrovirus packaging cells based on gibbon ape leukemia virus. J Virol 1991;65:2220—4.

[21] Parker LL, Do MT, Westwood JA, Wunderlich JR, Dudley ME, Rosenberg SA, et al. Expansion and characterization of T cells transduced with a chimeric receptor against ovarian cancer. Hum Gene Ther 2000;11:2377—87.

[22] Guidance for Industry USDoH, Human Services F, Drug Administration CfBE, Research. Supplemental guidance on testing for replication-competent retrovirus in retroviral vector-based gene therapy products and during follow-up of patients in clinical trials using retroviral vectors. Hum Gene Ther 2001;12:315—20.

[23] FDA. Testing of retroviral vector-based human gene therapy products for replication competent retrovirus during product manufacture and patient follow-up. 2018.

[24] Maude SL, Teachey DT, Porter DL, Grupp SA. CD19-targeted chimeric antigen receptor T-cell therapy for acute lymphoblastic leukemia. Blood 2015;125:4017—23.

[25] Savoldo B, Ramos CA, Liu E, Mims MP, Keating MJ, Carrum G, et al. CD28 costimulation improves expansion and persistence of chimeric antigen receptor-modified T cells in lymphoma patients. J Clin Investig 2011;121:1822—6.

[26] Grupp SA, Kalos M, Barrett D, Aplenc R, Porter DL, Rheingold SR, et al. Chimeric antigen receptor-modified T cells for acute lymphoid leukemia. N Engl J Med 2013;368:1509—18.

[27] Vander Heiden MG, Cantley LC, Thompson CB. Understanding the Warburg effect: the metabolic requirements of cell proliferation. Science 2009;324:1029–33.

[28] Goldman RD, Kaplan NO, Hall TC. Lactic dehydrogenase in human neoplastic tissues. Cancer Res 1964;24:389–99.

[29] Wolchok JD, Hoos A, O'Day S, Weber JS, Hamid O, Lebbe C, et al. Guidelines for the evaluation of immune therapy activity in solid tumors: immune-related response criteria. Clin Cancer Res 2009;15:7412–20.

[30] Schwartz LH, Litiere S, de Vries E, Ford R, Gwyther S, Mandrekar S, et al. RECIST 1.1-Update and clarification: from the RECIST committee. Eur J Cancer 2016;62:132–7.

[31] Hodi FS, Ballinger M, Lyons B, Soria JC, Nishino M, Tabernero J, et al. Immune-modified response evaluation criteria in solid tumors (imRECIST): refining guidelines to assess the clinical benefit of cancer immunotherapy. J Clin Oncol 2018;36:850–8.

[32] Eisenhauer EA, Therasse P, Bogaerts J, Schwartz LH, Sargent D, Ford R, et al. New response evaluation criteria in solid tumours: revised RECIST guideline (version 1.1). Eur J Cancer 2009;45:228–47.

[33] Watanabe H, Okada M, Kaji Y, Satouchi M, Sato Y, Yamabe Y, et al. [New response evaluation criteria in solid tumours-revised RECIST guideline (version 1.1)]. Gan To Kagaku Ryoho 2009;36:2495–501.

[34] Woodard HQ, Holodny E. A summary of the data of Mechanik on the distribution of human bone marrow. Phys Med Biol 1960;5:57–9.

[35] Cheson BD, Pfistner B, Juweid ME, Gascoyne RD, Specht L, Horning SJ, et al. Revised response criteria for malignant lymphoma. J Clin Oncol 2007;25:579–86.

[36] Cheson BD, Horning SJ, Coiffier B, Shipp MA, Fisher RI, Connors JM, et al. Report of an international workshop to standardize response criteria for non-Hodgkin's lymphomas. NCI Sponsored International Working Group. J Clin Oncol 1999;17:1244.

[37] Juweid ME. Utility of positron emission tomography (PET) scanning in managing patients with Hodgkin lymphoma. Hematol Am Soc Hematol Educ Program 2006;259–65:510–1.

[38] Juweid ME, Cheson BD. Positron-emission tomography and assessment of cancer therapy. N Engl J Med 2006;354:496–507.

CHAPTER 5

Challenges and Opportunities to Improve CAR T-Cell Therapy

CAR T-CELL EXHAUSTION

T-cell exhaustion has received great attention due to the success of checkpoint receptor blockade inhibitory drugs (CRB), that is, Opidova, Keytruda, and Ipilimumab. The CRB drugs function by reversing functional aspects of T-cell exhaustion. Thus, T-cell exhaustion has been at the heart of the pursuit of multibillion-dollar investment to identify new immunotherapy targets or to improve the existing CRB drugs. By definition, T-cell exhaustion in cancer refers to a process in which subset of tumor antigen-specific T cells suspend their killing activities after experiencing persistent antigenic activation through tumors (Fig. 5.1A) [2–7]. Exhaustion in tumor antigen-specific T cells is associated with altered functional, metabolic, and epigenetic state. Exhaustion is maintained due to checkpoint PD1/PDL1-derived inhibitory signaling, and due to aberrant activity of histone methyltransferases as well as DNA methyltransferases such as Dnmt3a [8]. Besides, several transcription factors that include among the others YY1, IRF4, and NFAT play important roles related to the metabolic regulation and inhibitory checkpoint receptor expression in exhausted T cells [7,9]. The reason why exhaustion develops is because it helps antigen-specific T cells to avoid generating autoimmune responses to persistent antigens. Exhausted T cells suspend their activities by engaging checkpoint inhibitory receptors especially PD1 with PD-L1 to directly counter the activating TCR and costimulatory signals. A second mechanism by which exhausted T cells counter the cues of harmful potentially autoimmune responses is by downregulating type I cytokines, for example, IL2. The reason being that autocrine IL2 can further exacerbate harmful autoimmune responses by delivering signal 3 upon engagement with high affinity trimeric IL2 receptor on antigen-specific T cells. The loss of IL2 and upregulation of immune checkpoint receptors, PD1, Lag3, Tim3, TIGIT represents crucial axes by which exhausted T cells sustain their inactivity against tumors [10].

Chimeric antigen receptor (CAR)-T cells are known to lose potency and in vivo persistence especially in solid cancers. Even with B-cell malignancies, for example, B-ALL, CAR T-cell-treated patients after having achieved a long-term remission, in some cases, as high as 90% [11], yet 30%–60% patients have ultimately relapsed [12]. The reason why CAR-T cells lose in vivo persistence and potency remains unknown. However, it is interesting to note that CAR-T cells incorporating CD28 costimulatory molecule have shown features consistent with features of exhaustion such as enhanced expression of PD1, Lag3, and Tim3, that is, upregulation of checkpoint receptor axis as well as loss of IL2, IFNγ, that is, cytokine axis. The perturbation of these two axes of exhaustion have been reported not only in the in vitro assays but also against tumor targets in the in vivo experiments (Fig. 5.1B) [13–16]. Most CAR-T clinical trials registered in https://clinicaltrials.gov/ propose to test or have been already testing second-generation CARs incorporating CD28 costimulatory molecule (Table 5.1). Therefore, it can be expected based on the new evidences [7,14,16] that CAR-T incorporating CD28 costimulatory molecule may be more prone to exhaustion via upregulation of checkpoint axis and downregulation of cytokine axis. Loss of IL2 production is one of the key features associated with exhausted T cells infiltrating solid cancers and also in chronic viral infections [6,17,18]. IL2 cytokine is crucial for generating destructive T-cell adaptive responses against tumors promoting regression of visceral metastasis as demonstrated in mouse models of sporadic cancer and in metastatic melanoma patients who received high doses of IL2 [19–23]. As a type I cytokine, IL2 plays pivotal role in clonal expansion and persistence of virus- and tumor-reactive T cells, and in their effector activity [19,23]. Therefore, loss of IL2 can cripple antigen-specific T-cell responses. As with the unmodified T cells, CAR-T cells generated to target solid cancers have shown features consistent with IL2 failure mediated inhibition of cancer-killing functions in vivo [13,21,24–26]. Therefore, reversing IL2 loss in CAR-modified T cells may reverse functional exhaustion and help maintaining cancer-killing

Basics of Chimeric Antigen Receptor (CAR) Immunotherapy. https://doi.org/10.1016/B978-0-12-819573-4.00005-3

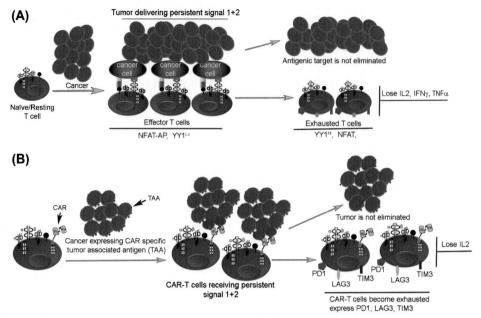

FIG. 5.1 Exhaustion in antigen-specific human T cells and CAR-T cells. Naïve or resting T cells when exposed to an immunogenic tumor differentiate into effector T cells. Several transcription factors are involved in maintaining effector phenotype of T cells, for example, NFAT-AP1 and YY1. The effector T cells produce effector molecules to eradicate cancer cells. However, in the persistent presence of tumor antigens, the effector T cells lose their effector activity via upregulation of checkpoint receptors and downregulation of effector cytokines, for example, IL2, IFNγ, and become exhausted **(A)**. A similar mechanism of exhaustion phenotype is observed in CAR-T cells responding to persistent presence of cognate tumor-associated antigens **(B)**. Delivery of persistent signal 1+2 play a crucial role in the rise of exhaustion phenotype in both antigen-specific unmodified and CAR-modified T cells.

activities [7]. Apart from IL2, IL7 is another important cytokine that is known to enhance survival and proliferation of T cells and for maintaining T-cell memory [27,28]. Therefore, the idea to use CAR-T therapy in combination with antiexhaustion checkpoint receptor blockade inhibitory drugs, for example anti-PD1 and anti-PDL1, and cytokine genes has gained significant attention recently. Adachi et al. demonstrated that tandem expression of IL7, chemokine ligand CCL19, and anti-CD20 CARs with 2A peptide sequence resulted in enhanced proliferation of CAR-T cells compared to anti-CD20 CAR alone when stimulated with anti-CD3 antibody in vitro or when cocultured with CD20 expressing mastocytoma cell line [29]. It remains to be seen if this particular approach provides any clinical benefits to the patients experiencing loss of CAR-T functions in vivo. It may be preferable to develop a system that could help CAR-T cells to first sense intrinsic loss of cytokines and then autonomously promote inducible IL2 or IL7 transgene expression. This approach can address loss of cytokine axis during CAR-T

exhaustion. As to addressing the upregulation of checkpoint axis, John et al. demonstrated that administrating anti-PD1 antibody along with anti-HER2-CD28 CAR T cells into HER2 transgenic mice implanted with HER2+ breast carcinoma cell lines caused significant tumor growth inhibition and also improved anti-HER2 CAR T-cell proliferation and activation [15]. Similarly, Burga et al. demonstrated that by combining anti-CEA.CD28.CAR with anti-PDL-1 antibody helped to inhibit PD1 (on CAR-T cell)/PDL1 (on liver MDSCs) interactions resulting in reduced liver metastasis in mice transplanted with MC38CEA tumor cells [30]. Several recently published papers have demonstrated that by infusing CD28.CARs with anti-PD1 checkpoint receptor blockade inhibitory antibody can improve in vivo persistence, effector cytokine production, and tumor cytotoxicity against solid cancers [14,31,32]. The anti-PD1 antibody can be delivered systemically into human patients receiving CAR-T cells. The timepoint at which anti-PD1 antibody can be delivered to patients must be determined experimentally and based on CAR-T

TABLE 5.1
List of CAR-T Clincial Trials Registered in https://clinicaltrials.gov/.

Target Antigen	Disease	CAR Signaling Domain	ClinicalTrial.gov Identifier	Clinical Center
CD19	B-CLL	CD28-CD3ζ	NCT00466531	MSKCC
CD19	B-ALL	CD28-CD3ζ	NCT01044069	MSKCC
CD19	Leukemia	CD28-CD3ζ	NCT01416974	MSKCC
CD19	Leukemia/lymphoma	CD28-CD3ζ	NCT00924326	NCI
CD19	Leukemia/lymphoma	CD28-CD3ζ	NCT01087294	NCI
CD19	Leukemia/lymphoma	CD28-CD3ζ versus CD3ζ	NCT00586391	BCM
CD19	B-NHL/CLL	CD28-CD3ζ versus CD3ζ	NCT00608270	BCM
CD19	Advanced B-NHL/CLL	CD28-CD3ζ versus CD3ζ	NCT00709033	BCM
CD19	ALL post-HSCT	CD28-CD3ζ	NCT00840853	BCM
CD19	Leukemia/lymphoma	CD137-CD3ζ	NCT01029366	UP
CD19	B-lymphoid malignancies	CD28-CD3ζ	NCT00968760	MDACC
CD19	B-lineage malignancies	CD28-CD3ζ	NCT01362452	MDACC
CD20	Mantle cell lymphoma/indolent B-NHL	CD28-CD137-CD3ζ	NCT00621452	FHCRC
PMSA	Prostate cancer	CD28-CD3ζ	NCT01140373	MSKCC
CEA	Breast cancer	CD28-CD3ζ	NCT00673829	RWMC
CEA	Colorectal cancer	CD28-CD3ζ	NCT00673322	RWMC
Her2/neu	Lung cancer	CD28-CD3ζ	NCT00889954	BCM
Her2/neu	Osteosarcoma	CD28-CD3ζ	NCT00902044	BCM
Her2/neu	Glioblastoma	CD28-CD3ζ	NCT01109095	BCM
Kappa light chain	B-NHL and B-CLL	CD28-CD3ζ versus CD3ζ	NCT00881920	BCM

Majority of studies propose to test CD28-CD3ζ CARs in their clincial trial protocols.
BCM, Baylor College of Medicine; *FHCRC*, Fred Hutchinson Cancer Research Center; *MDACC*, M.D. Anderson Cancer Center; *MSKCC*, Memorial Sloan-Kettering Cancer Center; *NCI*, National Cancer Institute; *RWMC*, Roger Williams Medical Center; *UP*, University of Pennsylvania.

dose response evaluations. It may be desirable to block PD1 checkpoint inhibitory signaling in CAR-T cells by developing cell intrinsic mechanisms. For example, by employing genetic engineering techniques, a PD1-dominant negative mutant expression vector can be inserted into CAR-T cells. The PD1-dominant negative mutant with deleted or mutated intracellular inhibitory domains will no longer be able to deliver inhibitory signaling. Moreover, the dominant negative mutant PD1 receptor interactions with PDL-1 will help fast saturating the total PD1 inhibitory signaling. Similarly, an inducible system can be designed in which PD1 specific shRNA can be inserted into CAR-T vector design.

The inducible anti-PD1 shRNA can be induced to express when effector activity of CAR-T cells begins to show decline. Cherkassky et al. successfully demonstrated that the dominant negative PD1 and PD1-specific shRNA can reverse functional exhaustion in mesothelin-specific CAR-T cells in the in vitro system as well in the in vivo orthotopic NSG mice that were implanted with human mesothelioma tumor cells [14]. Several novel genome-editing tools have been created recently that can precisely and efficiently edit gene sequences of the genome. One such genome-editing tool is CRISPR-Cas9 technology. The CRISPR-Cas9 technology is envisioned to be used for the therapeutic applications in humans to correct genetic disorders. The CRISPR-Cas9 technology can be applied in CAR therapy to silence checkpoint receptor inhibitory molecules, PD1, CTLA4, and other molecules driving exhaustion of CAR-T cells. The drawback with this approach may be generation of potential toxic autoimmune responses due to complete genomic deletion of checkpoint receptor inhibitory molecules, and a second drawback could be generation of adaptive immune responses against bacterially derived Cas9. The Cas9 is derived from *Staphylococcus aureus* and *Streptococcus pyogenes* strains. Interestingly, both Cas9-specific antibody and T cells have been detected in humans, indicating Cas9 could potentially induce antibody and T-cell-mediated responses when introduced in combination with CAR-T cells [33].

Several other approaches have been adopted to enhance potency of CARs, for example, via harnessing T memory stem cell properties, novel chemokine transgene expression, and by preventing aberrant activation-induced cell death. Memory T cells are rare subset of T cells in human body with huge potential to sustain persistence and generating antigen-specific memory. T memory stem cells possess huge self-renewal capacity and are primary precursor cells for generating long-lived memory [34]. However, due to their lower percentage in human peripheral blood, these rarely get modified with CARs; thus, the chances of generating a long-lived memory in CAR-T cells remain negligible. It is possible to transfer some of the properties of memory T cells to CAR-T cells via IL15 cytokine signaling. IL15 like IL2 signals through the common cytokine receptor γ-chain and is crucial for memory T-cell generation as well as NK and CD8 T-cell expansion [35–37]. Moreover, IL15 is being tested as an immunotherapy target in clinical trials either alone or in combination with TILs, besides IL15 has been shown to be important for suppressing cancerous growth through generation of distinct set of innate lymphocytes that demonstrated potent cytolytic activity against tumor cells in spontaneous murine mammary tumor model [38–40]. Interestingly, IL15 functions in a unique manner, different from other soluble cytokines that are secreted locally into the medium; IL15 is exported on the surface of IL15-producing cells especially dendritic cells bound to IL15Rα in a process termed as *transpresentation*. IL15 in complex with IL15Rα is presented to NK and CD8 memory T cells where it is recognized by IL15/IL2 receptor βγ chain [41]. IL2 and IL15 share the common βγ receptor chains. Hurton et al. by harnessing the unique transpresentation mechanism of IL15/IL15Rα were able to demonstrate the transfer of T memory stem cell like properties into anti-CD19 CAR T cells generating memory responses along with potent toxicity against CD19$^+$ B-cell cancers [42]. Hurton et al. coexpressed gene sequences encoding IL15/IL15Rα (membrane bound IL15) together with second-generation CD19-CAR using sleeping beauty system. The membrane bound IL15 signaling (signal 3) activated STAT5-mediated gene transcription program and generated T stem cell memory phenotype CD45RO$^-$CCR7$^+$ in anti-CD19 CAR modified T cells, besides helped these to maintain potent and persistent antitumor cytotoxicity (Fig. 5.2). Similarly, the chemokine receptor genes have also been tested to enhance CAR T-cell tumor trafficking. For example, CCR4 has been expressed to enhance CD30-CAR trafficking to target Hodgkin's Lymphoma [43].

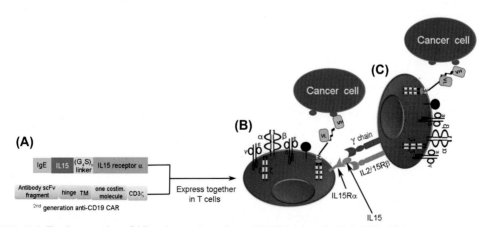

FIG. 5.2   T cell expressing a CAR and a membrane bound IL15Rα tethered with IL15 **(A–B)** that upon interaction with IL15Rβ and common gamma chain (γc) also shared by IL2 receptors among other cytokines **(C)**. The IL15Rα-IL15 interactions with IL15/IL2βγ-chain triggers signaling and gene activation program in CAR-T cells conferring a memory T stem cell phenotype. The attaining of memory T stem cell phenotype can help generating long-lived memory in CAR-T cells.

Addressing limitation of CAR-T survival in vivo. Several second-generation CAR-modified T cells appeared to undergo programmed cell death resembling activation-induced cell death in vitro and in vivo in tumor-bearing host [21,44]. The CAR T-cell apoptosis has been reported to undergo both intrinsic and extrinsic apoptotic cell death pathways triggered by IL2 depletion and upregulation of Fas/FasL death receptor ligands interactions [21,44]. To improve the overall survival of CAR T cells by enhancing resistance against apoptosis, the genes encoding BCL_{XL} and $FLIP_L$ have been incorporated into second generations CARs. BCL_{XL} is a $BCL2$ homolog of one of the two splice variants of $BCL2L1$ gene, the other being the shorter form BCL-X$_S$ [45]. The BCL$_{XL}$ is a prosurvival protein, which is involved in preventing intrinsic cell death pathway by sequestering BH3-only proteins, BAX and BAK. The BAX and BAK are involved in sensing cell death signals and promoting mitochondrial membrane leakage causing mitochondrial membrane permeability transition [46,47]. BCL$_{XL}$ is, thus, crucial for interrupting procaspase activation. Moreover, in the T cells, BCL$_{XL}$ protein expression is enhanced by CD28 costimulation through PI3K-mTOR signaling pathway that helps through intrinsic mechanisms to prevent apoptosis caused by either Fas cross-linking or IL2 withdrawal [48–50]. FLIPs [FADD like interleukin-1β-converting enzyme like protease (FLICE/caspase-8)-inhibitory protein] are involved in apoptosis in extrinsic cell death pathway triggered by Fas/FasL interaction at the surface of activated T cells. Two splice variants of $FLIP$ are expressed in humans, a long and a short transcript, FLIP$_L$ and FLIP$_s$ respectively. Both isoforms share structural homology with procaspase 8 but lack catalytic activity that allows these to bind to the death inducing silencing complex that among the others is composed of FADD/TRADD and initiator caspase 8. Their binding prevents activation of initiator caspase 8, thus, helps to blocks Fas and TNF RI-induced extrinsic cell death pathways [51,52]. Charo et al. examined the effect of FLIP$_L$ overexpression in activated primary T cells and melanoma antigen-specific T cells, their results support that FLIP$_L$ can prevent activation induced cell death (AICD), and promote survival of T cells. However, FLIP$_L$-modified T cells were unable to sustain cytokine production [53]. These data support that CAR-T cells modified with antiapoptotic genes could help these to resist cell death and enhance persistence at the tumor sites. The unpublished data from our laboratory have demonstrated that expressing BCL_{XL} and $FLIP_L$ transgenes in tandem with CEA tumor antigen-specific CARs can prevent IL2 withdrawal and Fas-mediated apoptosis of CEA-CAR T cells. These measures helped CAR T-cell survival and maintained superior cancer cytotoxicity (Balkhi MY and Junghans RP, unpublished data).

CONTROLLING ANTIGEN ESCAPE IN CAR-T CELLS

The CAR-T therapy results especially those obtained with second-generation CARs that incorporate costimulatory molecule have demonstrated tremendous success in eradicating CD19$^+$ B-cell malignancies [54–56]. Perhaps CD19 as a choice of tumor antigen for CAR targeting made it very successful because CD19 is a B-cell identity marker and its expression is maintained from early B-cell lineage to mature B-cell stages [57]. Its expression is maintained in bone barrow recirculating B cells, marginal, and follicular B cells [58–60]. CD19 expression on various B-cell types and during different B-cell malignancies marks it best choice for CAR targeting. However, as discussed earlier, despite being almost perfect target, anti-CD19 CARs have encountered problems in vivo. Several B-ALL patients have relapsed after achieving long-term remission [12]. Apart from the CD19-CAR T exhaustion [13], antigen escape may be one of the underlying mechanism for the loss of anti-CD19 CAR potency in vivo. Antigen escape refers to the process in which tumor cells reduce targeted tumor antigens or produce mutant variants of targeted tumor antigen to escape immune recognition [61]. For example, CD19$^+$ B-cell cancers under selection pressure from anti-CD19 CAR targeting evolve CD19$^-$ B-cell cancer variants helping these to evade CAR-T-mediated killings. The development of CD19$^-$ B-cell cancers has been reported to occur in 10%–28% of ALL and CLL patients after having received CD19 CAR-T infusions [62–65]. Even in the in vitro essays, the phenomenon of antigen escape has been observed. The targeting of HER2 tumor-associated antigen on glioblastoma cell lines have led to rise of HER2-tumor variants [66]. Antigen escape is not restricted to tumors only, antigen escape variants can develop in response to antiviral drugs and vaccines developed to treat HIV1 infections [67,68].

Targeting antigen escape. Bispecific CARs have been created to counter antigen escape by targeting two tumor-associated antigens in tandem. This is elaborated here. Apart from CD19, CD22 and BCMA are two B-cell lineage markers that have been used for CAR targeting in ALL and multiple myeloma, respectively [69–71]. CD22 is a membrane immunoglobulin protein that has been reported to be expressed predominantly on

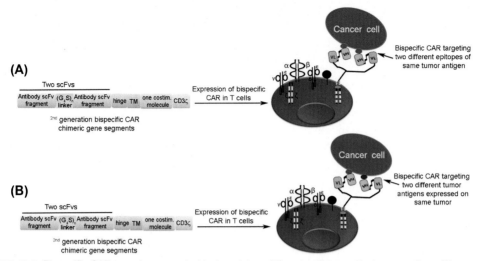

FIG. 5.3 Bispecific CARs can be generated to target two different epitopes of a tumor antigen **(A)** or two different tumor-associated antigens expressed on same tumor **(B)** or two different tumors (not shown). The two antibody scFvs in a bispecific CAR are usually separated through a glycine-rich linker.

B cells and appears to negatively regulate B-cell receptor signaling through their intracellular tyrosine inhibitory motifs that serve to recruit SH2 homology phosphatases, SHP1 and SHP2 [72,73]. CD19/CD22-bispecific CARs have been created to block antigen escape and eliminate mixed CD19+CD20+ or CD19+CD20− or CD19− CD20+ cancer variant phenotypes [74]. The concept of bispecific CARs is both practical and feasible. The bispecific CARs can be created to target two different epitopes of the same tumor antigen (Fig. 5.3A) or two different tumor antigens expressed on the same cancer, for example, CD19/CD22, CEA/TAG72, or PSMA/PSCA (Fig. 5.3B). The two antibody scFv fragments in a bispecific CAR may be separated by glycine serine linkers, for example, (glycin$_4$ serine)$_2$ or (glycin$_4$ serine)$_4$ [74−76]. The utility of such bispecific CARs is immense as in case of CD19 or CD22 antigen loss, CAR can still target either of the two antigens. Even a bispecific CAR can be created to target two totally different cell-type-specific antigens. For example, a bispecific CAR was created expressing anti-HER2/Neu+ plus anti-CD19. The HER2/Neu is not expressed in B-cell lineage whereas CD19 is not expressed on epithelial cancers such as breast cancer. Yet, conceptually it is possible to create CARs targeting several different antigens. However, the utility of bispecific CARs targeting two different lineage antigens may be limited unless patient suffers from two different lineage restricted cancers. Overall, creating a bispecific CAR may be more practical than simply mixing two CAR-T products such as anti-CD19 CAR and anti-CD20 CAR followed by

their transduction into patient T cells or simply pooling two different monospecific CAR-T products and then injecting CAR-T mixture into patients. In the former method, the expression and stoichiometry of two CARs in the same T cells cannot be controlled whereas injecting two separate CARs into patients will involve investing double the efforts in manufacturing and developing CAR infusion clinical protocols. Nevertheless, the combinatorial approach has shown some benefits in eradicating glioblastoma tumor cell line U373 in vitro assays as well as xenograft glioblastoma tumors in mice [66]. Overall, bispecific CARs represent valuable tool for tumor targeting and to overcome the challenge of tumor antigen escape.

MONITORING CAR-T PERSISTENCE IN VIVO

After CAR-T cells have been infused into patients, the challenge is to examine their persistence, quantitating their survival and growth, and determining if CAR-T cells have trafficked to tumors. Even more challenging is to assess if CAR-T cells have generated memory responses in recipient patients. All these measures can help to predict patient's response to CAR therapy. However, at present, techniques to monitor noninvasively the CAR T-cell trafficking to tumors and in vivo persistence are not available. Therefore, it is essential to design CARs in such a way so that these functions can be measured and evaluated. Some of these functions can be measured if CAR-T cells are cloned to express a tag or a fluorescent marker. The marker or a tag can be followed in vivo through fluorescent imaging or utilized to analyze through flow cytometry to assess persistence, proliferation, trafficking, and any potential phenotype changes. Recently, a reporter gene technology was used to image CAR-T cells in vivo. Anti-IL13Rα2 CAR in combination with herpes simplex virus type 1 thymidine kinase fusion gene (HSV1-tk) was tested in vivo. The *HSV1-tk* fusion gene included *HSV1-tk* suicidal gene and constitutively expressing positron emission tomography (PET) reporter gene with a purpose to monitor tumor trafficking and persistence. The anti-IL13Rα2- HSV1-tk CAR was ectopically expressed into CD8 T cells using electroporation and subsequently injected intratumorally into stage IV glioblastoma patient. Three weeks later, the patient undergo whole body PET scanning to detect infused CAR-T cells constitutively expressing PET reporter gene. The CAR-T cells were visualized in the body using PET reporter probe 9-[4-[^{18}F]fluoro-3-(hydroxymethyl)butyl]guanine ([^{18}F]FHBG) that was injected into patient through i.v. line [77,78]. Upon superimposing PET images with MRI images of the affected organ, the CAR T-cell trafficking and persistence could be visualized and corroborated with the antitumor responses. This technology apart from some issues with background and nonspecific accumulation of [^{18}F]FHBG in tissues provides an excellent tool for monitoring CAR T-cell persistence in vivo.

CAR T-cell phenotype changes. Polychromatic flow cytometry-based techniques offer best choice to characterize CAR-T phenotype changes especially CAR memory phenotypes in vivo. CARs expressing Histidine or myc tag or fluorescent genes encoding eGFP or mCherry protein [79,80] can be very useful in characterizing CAR-T cell phenotypes. The fluorescent probes and tags can allow straight forward estimation of percent modification of T cells, besides these can prove useful for CAR-T isolation from blood, bone marrow, and resected tumors. The isolated CAR-T cells can be processed for cellular and molecular analyses such as memory phenotype assessment, proliferation capacity, and assessment of their effector functions including cytokine and chemokine production [81]. Novel CAR-T tumor targeting approaches combined with provisions for monitoring CAR-T persistence and tumor cytotoxicity have recently been demonstrated in vitro and in vivo murine models. One such approach has been fluorochrome-based adaptors designed by chemist Philip Low, PhD, and doctoral student Yong-Gu Lee of Purdue University, Indianapolis. They have synthesized so-called adaptors. These adapters are fusion molecules that express on one side a fluorescein isothiocyanate (FITC) molecule and on other side

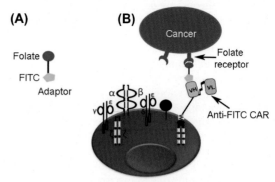

FIG. 5.4 The fluorochrome-based adaptors for CAR-mediated targeting of tumors. **(A)** A FITC fluorochrome-conjugated adaptor. These adapters are fusion molecules that express on one side a FITC molecule and other side a high affinity tumor-associated antigen ligand such as folate that binds to folate receptor α (FRα). **(B)** Anti-FITC CAR targeting a cancer cell through FITC adaptor. When anti-FITC CARs and FITC-conjugated folate adaptors are infused into tumor-bearing host. The adaptors will bind to the folate receptor-α expressed on the tumors. The anti-FITC CARs then target FITC adaptors bound to folate receptor-α allowing CARs to gain access to tumors **(A−B)**.

a high affinity tumor-associated antigen ligand such as folate that binds to folate receptor α (FRα), which is overexpressed in several cancers including ovarian, breast, and lung [82]. Lee and Low designed anti-FITC CAR, which is very less cumbersome when compared to designing tumor antigen-specific CARs. The anti-FITC CAR and adaptor were infused into tumor-bearing mice. The adaptors were able to bind to the folate receptors expressed by the tumors in vivo. The anti-FITC CAR targeted the folate receptor bound FITC adaptor that allows CARs to gain access to tumors inducing tumor killings (Fig. 5.4A,B) [83]. The advantage of having an FITC-conjugated adaptor is that it allows visualization of CAR-mediated tumor attack. However, one of the caveats of the approach is dependence on the adaptors for tumor targeting. It remains to be seen if adaptors can maintain binding with tumor antigens long enough to allow significant tumor lysis.

TOXICITIES ASSOCIATED WITH CAR THERAPY AND MANAGEMENT OF THOSE TOXICITIES

Majority of CARs generated to date are designed to target tumor-associated self-antigens. Therefore, some form of on-target/off-tumor toxicities especially autoimmune responses may be expected. In addition,

CAR-T cells in "theory" are designed to bind to the tumor antigens with optimal-binding specificities. Therefore, CAR-T-tumor antigen reactions are expected to induce proliferation, activation, and production of effector and proinflammatory cytokines. The kinetics of cytokines released by CARs in vivo cannot be accurately predicted; therefore, potential of cytokine-related toxicities may be an expected outcome of on-target/on-tumor reactions. Moreover, the necrotic tumor cargo left as a result of CAR T-cell-mediated tumor lysis can potentially lead to complement activation and cumulative proinflammatory responses referred to as tumor lysis syndrome due to macrophage activation and subsequent mediator releases such as IP10, IL1, IL6, and MIP1α [84]. Overall, the on-target/off-tumor-related toxicities, cytokine release syndrome and certain neurological events have emerged as major toxicity risks with CAR therapy.

The Cytokine Release Syndrome

Cytokine release syndrome (CRS) has been a consistent occurrence in CAR-therapy clinical trials [33,54,85]. The CRS can be mild (grade 1−2), moderate (grade 3), and severe (grades 4−5) that potentially can be life threatening [1,84]. Some of the common clinical symptoms observed in patients due to CAR-T-related CRS may range from flu like symptoms to fever, chills, headache, fatigue, myalgias, hypotension, hypoxia, dyspnea, tachycardia, vascular leak syndrome, acute rental failure, cardiorespiratory distress, multiple organ failure, and death [24,84,86]. The CRS observed with CAR therapy can be more severe when compared to similar type of syndromes observed with TILs or TCR therapy, the reason could be that the autologous TILs or TCRs react with the cognate antigens in their natural binding specificity as they do not rely on synthetic antigen-binding domains whereas artificial antigen-binding domains designed in CARs can bind with altered affinities that cannot be accurately predicted. Therefore, CRS is observed not only with CARs but also with other cancer targeting synthetic antibodies such as CD19/CD3-bispecific BiTE antibody blinatumomab [86,87]. The common inflammatory cytokines elevated during CRS include IFNγ, TNFα, IL6, IL8, IL10, sIL2Rα, MCP1, MIP1α, MIP1β, and markers of systemic inflammation, C-reactive protein (CRP), and ferritin. The IL6, CRP, and ferritin levels rise dramatically in patients experiencing severe form of CRS. The cytokine levels in patients receiving CAR-T therapy are assessed from the serum using either an ELISA or most commonly now high throughput multiplex ELISA technology [84,88]. It is not unconceivable to relate some of the CRS symptoms

directly to the cytokines, for example, TNFα apart from exerting antitumor effect is an inducer of hypotension, fatigue, and nausea [89]. Similarly, IFNγ is an inducer of fever, chills, fatigue, and granulocytopenia [90,91]. It is interesting to note that patients presented with severe forms of CRS especially in ALL often presented with high tumor burden and more CAR-T positive effector T cells responses indicating a correlation between CRS and productive tumor responses [54,85]. Curiously, no correlation between tumor burden and CRS was noted in CLL patients treated with CD19-CAR indicating that correlation between CRS and tumor responses may be tumor antigen specific [92]. The clinical features observed in CRS share many similarities with macrophage activation syndrome (MAS)/hemophagocytic lymphohistiocytosis (HLH) [93]. There are two forms of HLH, primary and secondary. The primary HLH in children is caused by rare germline mutation in genes involved in cytolytic granule exocytosis; whereas, secondary HLH also known as MAS believed to be nonhereditary is often associated with infections, autoimmune disorders, and cancer [94,95]. HLH is characterized by diffuse infiltration of histiocytes into vital organs. Histiocytes show hemophagocytic activity and patients present with abnormal immune activation [96]. Apart from the common clinical symptoms observed between HLH/MAS and CRS, those ranging from mild symptoms to severe including multiorgan damage, IL10, IL6, and IFNγ are the most important cytokines that are elevated in MAS/HLH [55,95]. The elevated levels of these cytokines after CAR-T infusion indicate macrophage activation and potential role of macrophages in driving some aspect of CRS [55,86].

Neurotoxicity has emerged as an unexpected feature associated with CAR therapy. Adverse neurological events have been observed in association with CRS or immediately after the development of CRS, and following the resolution of CRS or without any CRS [62,97,98]. Neurotoxicity has been predominantly observed in patients receiving anti-CD19 CAR therapy but not without an exception, as reports also exist of CLL patients achieving complete remission with CD19-CAR therapy without developing any CRS or neurological events [97,99]. The complications arising due to neurotoxicity range from mild to severe. The neurologic adverse events can be graded according to National Cancer Institute Common Toxicity Criteria for Adverse Events (NCI CTCAE v5.0) [100]. Delirium and seizures, confusion that may progress to deficiency in communication, aphasia, obtunded, cerebral edema, choreoathetosis, and fatal intracranial hemorrhage are some of the manifestations of neurologic toxicities observed with CD19-CARs [33,88,101]. These neurological complications may become severe requiring intubation and mechanical ventilation. However, some of these neurological complications are reversible. The underlying mechanism causing the neurological disturbances is presently unclear. Some recent data have suggested that neurotoxicity especially cerebral edema could be due to direct result of CRS triggering endothelial activation and blood brain barrier (BBB) permeability and leakage of systemic inflammatory cytokines including IFNγ into cerebrospinal fluid [97]. Recently, first nonhuman primate rhesus macaque (RM) model of neurotoxicity was developed. An infusion of anti-CD20 CAR following cyclophosphamide lymphodepletion induces CRS and neurotoxicity. The neurotoxicity in the RM model seem to be associated with very high levels of IL6, IL2, GM-CSF, and VEGF levels in the cerebrospinal fluid (CSF). Moreover, cellular infiltrates including anti-CD20 CAR and unmodified T cells appear to have accumulated in the CSF and brain parenchyma [102].

Management of cytokine release syndrome and neurologic toxicity. Management of CAR-T-related CRS and CAR-T-related encephalopathy syndrome (CRES) forms essential component of contingency protocols in CAR therapy. The treatment options to control CRS have been related to the severity of CRS. The mild forms of CRS that present with no major clinical toxicities may require no more than observation and modest forms of routine medical treatment, whereas patients presented with severe CRS require urgent medical intervention. Therefore, for the better clinical management of CRS, a better understanding of CRS biology is needed. Moreover, robust diagnostic criteria must be adopted to confidently diagnose CRS from other unrelated comorbidities. In addition, predictive models must be developed to provide probability of patients developing severe CRS [84]. In general, three forms of treatment have been applied to control severe CRS/MAS. These include steroids, anti-IL6 receptor monoclonal antibody (tocilizumab), anti-CD25 (anti-IL2Rα) monoclonal antibody (daclizumab), and inhibitors, for example, anti-IL1R inhibitor (anakinra) [95]. Administration of high doses of steroids to patients presented with severe CRS can lead to rapid control of fever, lowering of serum cytokines levels, and reversal of other clinical symptoms. However, steroid treatments have also resulted in loss of CD19-CAR T-cell proliferation and persistence that can severely compromise tumor eradication [101]. In two separate studies, Brentjens et al. and Grupp et al. [54,55] did not report any loss of CD19-CAR-T cell activity in

patients who had been on steroids. Nevertheless, potential adverse effect imposed by steroids on CAR-T functions needed to be evaluated. Tocilizumab have also led to the rapid reversal of clinical symptoms associated with CRS; however, in contrast to steroids, tocilizumab did not adversely affect persistence and expansion of CAR-T cells in patients [55,101]. Tocilizumab is humanized monoclonal antibody that binds to membrane bound and soluble IL6R blocking IL6 binding to its receptors. IL6 exerts its biological functions by binding to the membrane bound IL6R and soluble IL6R (sIL6R) via classical and trans-signaling pathways, respectively. The IL6 ligand binding to IL6Rα receptor leads to recruitment and homodimerization of gp130 to form tetrameric receptor complex. The ligand binding leads to the activation of gp130-associated kinases, Jak1, Jak2, and Tyk2, and the tyrosine residues within cytoplasmic tail of gp130 become phosphorylated to serve as docking sites for STAT1 and STAT3. Subsequently, STAT1 and STAT3 become phosphorylated, dimerize, and translocate to nucleus to activate IL6-mediated gene transcription program [103]. IL6 regulates many biological functions apart from the innate and adaptive immune functions. IL6 is important for protecting cardiovascular and neural functions, and bone homeostasis. Its immune functions include promoting survival of T cells, differentiation of naïve T cells to effector Th17 cells, and inhibition of TGF-β-driven inducible Treg cell development [104]. Because tocilizumab essentially blocks IL6 receptor signaling and shuts off its biological functions that begs explanation whether cell-type-specific blocking of IL6 receptor signaling employing JAK kinase inhibitors [105] may be more useful as long-term implications of systemic blocking of IL6R on CAR-T functions remain unknown. Fortunately, tocilizumab has been tested in large phase I–III clinical trials for the treatment of juvenile idiopathic arthritis (JIA) and adult rheumatoid arthritis (RA), no major toxicities were reported except marked increase in liver enzymes and mild neutropenia and thrombocytopenia [106–109]. Besides, tocilizumab is an FDA and European Medicines Agency approved drug for the treatment of RA and JIA in patients above 2 years of age [95]. As to the source of IL6 in CRS, macrophages and monocyte most likely secrete IL6 during tumor attack [106,110]. However, there are other cell types that also secrete IL6 including T cells, monocytes, dendritic cells, endothelial cells, and osteocytes. The identification of major source of IL6 production during CRS will help developing cell-type-specific blockade of IL6R signaling.

Apart from IL6R blockade, several other soluble cytokine receptor agonists have been tested to treat

CRS. Among which, sIL2Rα agonist daclizumab (Zenapax, Roche, Germany) has shown potential benefits in controlling abnormal immune activation [111]. It is interesting to note that sIL2Rα level increases significantly in patients experiencing CRS after receiving CD19-CAR T-cell infusion. A similar rise of sIL2Rα was also reported in HLH. The daclizumab would essentially downmodulate the sIL2Rα activity by neutralizing it. It was successfully applied to treat the child with HLH [111]. One of the major drawbacks associated with using anti-IL2R agonists may be its direct effect on CAR T-cell survival and functions. IL2 cytokine is crucial for destructive T-cell responses against tumors and promoting regression of visceral metastasis as shown in mouse models of sporadic cancer and in metastatic melanoma patients receiving high doses of IL2 [19–23]. Therefore, extreme caution must be adopted when applying interventions that affect IL2 functions. In addition to IL6 and IL-2Rα, IL1 blockade has also resulted in resolution of CRS in mice studies [110,112]. Norelli et al. utilizing humanized NSG mouse model with reconstituted human hematopoiesis system demonstrated that monocytes to be a major source of IL1, and IL1 release preceded IL6 indicating that IL1 may be the primary source for initiating CRS. They further demonstrated that administration of anakinra, which is an anti-human IL1 receptor (IL1Rα) antagonist, was effective in protecting mice from CRS-related mortality. In another study, Giavridis et al. utilizing SCID-beige mice to study CAR T-related CRS reported that myeloid cells play a greater role in CRS pathogenesis. They demonstrated that CAR T-cell tumor attack apart from macrophages help to activate and re-cruit myeloid cells prompting IL1, IL6, and nitric oxide (NO) release. Remarkably, by applying anakinra to blockade IL-1 receptor signaling, they could also abolish CRS-related mortalities [112].

Management of neurotoxicity. We have only recently begun to understand the molecular and cellular mechanisms causing the neurological symptoms with CAR therapy, and with the establishment of first nonhuman primate RM model of CAR-T, CRS, and neurotoxicity [102]. The model should allow us to understand if the neurotoxicity with CAR therapy has a separate pathophysiology or merely a bystander effect of CRS triggering endothelial activation and BBB permeability allowing CAR-T and unmodified T-cell infiltration and flow of systemic proinflammatory cytokines into cerebrospinal fluid [97,101,113]. It is interesting to note that even though patients demonstrate neurological events, the brain scan images often turn out unremarkable. Except in the fatal cases, neurological events are reversible and self-limiting. The Hematopoietic Stem Cell Transplantation, Subgroup of the Pediatric Acute Lung Injury and Sepsis Investigators, and the MD Anderson Cancer Center CAR T-Cell Therapy-Associated Toxicity guidelines as well as the previously published guidelines for CRES management in children and adults have provided comprehensive mechanisms for monitoring and management of CRES [98,114]. Some of the key recommendations proposed for monitoring and management of CRES are listed:

1. Perform CRES grading every 12 hours. If clinical status alters, performing more frequent CRES grading is recommended.
2. Ensuring anti-IL6 therapy is available.
3. Levetiracetam drug (10 mg/kg, up to a maximum of 500 mg per dose), every 12 hours for 30 days after CAR T-cell infusion in patients if experience seizure.
4. A baseline neurology exams employing electroencephalography, MRI of the brain and spinal cord is recommended for patients with a history of seizures or underlying CNS diseases.
5. If cranial pressure increases with no evidence of cerebral edema consider administering acetazolamide 15 mg/kg (maximum 1000 mg) i.v. followed by 8–12 mg/kg (maximum 1000 mg) i.v. every 12 hours.
6. If intracranial pressure increases with conclusive evidences of cerebral edema on imaging scans, consider using high-dose of corticosteroids along with hyperosmolar therapy and if patient presents with Ommaya reservoir draining of CSF is recommended. Moreover, neurosurgery consultations must be considered for further contingency.

On-Target/Off-Tumor Toxicity

CARs targeting tumor-associated self-antigens may invariably cause destruction of healthy tissues expressing the targeted antigen. For example, CD19−CAR apart from targeting malignant B cells will most likely also target normal cells of CD19+ B-cell lineage that could lead to B-cell depletion and hypogammaglobulinemia [86,88]. The third-generation Herceptin-based human epidermal growth factor receptor 2 (HER2-CAR) developed to specifically target metastatic colon carcinoma have resulted in severe toxicity and death [115,116], apparently due to CRS triggered by CAR targeting of ERBB2 on lung epithelial tissues. HER2/neu is a tyrosine kinase receptor encoded by the *ERBB2* gene. HER2 overexpression is associated with several cancers such as ovarian, stomach, lung, uterus, and salivary duct carcinoma [117,118], but it is also expressed at low level on healthy tissues [119]. Similarly, anti-GD2

CAR developed to treat neuroblastoma resulted in fatal neurotoxicity [120], apparently due to massive infiltration of CAR-T into brain tissues leading to neuronal damage. The disialoganglioside glycolipid (GD2) is highly expressed on neuroblastoma cells but also normally on a developing and adult brain. The fatal neurotoxicity observed with anti-GD2 CAR was unexpected as preclinical studies in mice have shown specific targeting of GD$^+$ human neuroblastoma xenograft. As a further proof of prevalence of on-target/off-tumor toxicity with CARs, in a phase I trial targeting metastatic renal cell carcinoma carbonic anhydrase IX (CAIX) tumor-associated antigen with first-generation anti-CAIX CAR resulted in significant liver toxicities in some patients necessitating to halt the treatment. The bile duct epithelium biopsy examination revealed low-level CAIX expression and unmodified T cells and anti-CAIX CAR-modified T-cell infiltration [25]. These few examples demonstrate that despite the selection of perfect tumor associated antigen, the CAR targeting of tumor-associated self-antigens can impose significant risk of off-tumor toxicity that may not be visible in preclinical models. Therefore, to avoid the off-target toxicity CARs have been modified with suicide genes such as herpes simplex virus-thymidine kinase (*HSV-TK*) as well as caspase 9 (*iCasp9*) transgene safety-switch. The cloning of caspase 9 (*iCasp9*) transgene safety-switch with GD2-CAR allows destruction of disproportionally activated melanoma antigen-specific CARs T cells in preclinical studies [121,122]. The inducible expression of iCasp9 can be triggered by the administration of inhibitor drug, AP1903. However, these inducible artificial transgenes may not be enough to prevent the damage caused by the CAR targeting of vital tissues. Therefore, the choice of tumor antigen for CAR targeting remains the single most important factor in achieving tumor antigen-specific killings and avoiding on-target/off-tumor toxicity. How to achieve a tumor antigen-specific killing and at the same time avoid damage to healthy tissue? One way to achieve that could be isolating and characterizing unique tumor antigens. However, isolating and characterizing unique tumor antigens can be technically challenging. To overcome the challenge of mining unique tumor specific antigens, number of labs have focused on whole-exome sequencing and single-cell RNA-seq analysis combined with proteomic technology to identify novel tumor antigens [123−126]. These powerful new technologies is expected to help designing tumor-specific CARs, which are expected to greatly diminish off-tumor toxicities [127−130]. Similarly, cancer testis antigens that are only expressed in germline cells or thymic medullary epithelium but can get reexpressed in cancers offer

novel choices for generating tumor antigen-specific CARs [131]. Accordingly, NY-ESO-1 cancer testis antigen has been utilized for CAR targeting of multiple myeloma and neuroblastoma, and has already been successfully tested in preclinical animal models [132,133]. Apart from the choice of tumor antigens for CAR targeting, CAR structural domains can also influence antigen affinity binding that can hugely influence CAR functions [13]. Several other novel ideas have been recently tested with the intention of increasing precise CAR targeting of tumor antigens and minimizing off-tumor toxicities. A powerful combinatorial approach involving CAR targeting of two separate tumor antigens has been reported. In this combinatorial approach CAR recognition of one tumor antigen can lead to inducible expression and activation of a second CAR. The first CAR probes the tumor antigens that is followed by precise retargeting of tumor antigens with second CAR. Roybal et al. engineered a synthetic notch receptor. The synthetic notch receptor is composed of scFv ectodomain, a transmembrane domain, and a notch intracellular domain containing artificial transcription factor. The synthetic notch receptor intracellular domain is generated by replacing notch intracellular domain with artificial transcription factor domain. Synthetic notch receptor intracellular domains are without any conventional CAR costimulatory and CD3ζ signaling domains. The choice of using synthetic notch receptor for orthogonal signaling marks an excellent choice. Notch receptors and ligands are expressed in T cells where it is required for T-cell effector functions [134]. Besides, notch receptors are single-pass transmembrane protein composed of well-defined notch extracellular domain (NECD), a transmembrane domain (TM), and notch intracellular domain (NICD). NECD interaction with Delta-like or Jagged family ligand induce NICD cleavage from TM and NECD. In mammals, γ-secretase cleaves NICD from TM, and NICD subsequently translocates to the nucleus where it forms a transcription factor complex with CBF1/Su(H)/Lag-1 (CSL) that binds and activates notch target genes [135]. Roybal et al. replaced *NECD* of notch receptor with single-chain variable fragment of anti-CD19 antibody. In addition, they also replaced the intracellular *NICD* domain with artificial transcription factor domain, that is, *GAL4DBD-VP64* or *TetR-VP64*. Upon ligand binding, that is, CD19 antigen with synthetic notch receptor, orthogonal transcription factor gets cleaved from the TM. The cleaved orthogonal transcription factor like NICD translocates to the nucleus and activates the transcription of second CAR transgene, that is, antimesothelin second-generation CAR, whose promoter activation is placed under the control of

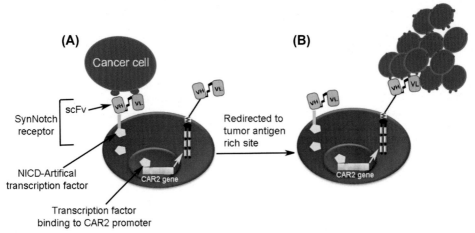

FIG. 5.5 Diagram of a synthetic notch receptor CAR sensing the tumor antigen and then through intracellular notch signaling pathway inducing the expression of second CAR. CAR-1 contains scFv generated to target tumor-associated antigen is fused with a synthetic notch receptor (SynNotch receptor) **(A)**. The scFv fused to SynNotch binding with a cognate tumor-associated antigen triggers proteolysis in the notch intracellular domain (NICD). The NICD domains are swapped with an artificial transcription factor. The NICD-transcription factor domain translocates to the nucleus where it binds to the promoter element of a second CAR (CAR-1). The NICD-transcription factor binding to the promoter of CAR-2 leads to the transcription and translation of CAR-2. The CAR-2 contains all domains of a conventional CAR. The CAR-1 senses the tumor antigens and sends a signal for the CAR-2 expression. The dual mechanism of tumor sensing and targeting can help minimizing the risk of off-tumor toxicities besides helping CARs redirected to tumors **(B)**.

synthetic notch-induced transcription factor. The second CAR is constructed to express all the components of a conventional CAR [136,137]. The synthetic notch receptor platform provides powerful tool to confer inbuilt antigen-sensing capabilities to CARs that can help redirecting CARs to target tumor antigen-rich environment and limit toxic off-target responses (Fig. 5.5A,B). One of the reasons why this technology can greatly minimize but may not completely eliminate on-target/off-tumor toxicities is because it allows CARs first to probe and sense tumor antigen without actually mounting tumor attack. Once the first CAR senses tumor antigen and sends signal to the promoter of second CAR to activate its transcription. There is a lag period before second CAR can get expressed and recognize tumor antigen. This mechanism can redirect CARs to access tumor antigen-rich environment and enhance in vivo persistence.

ALLOGENEIC CARS

The CAR therapy currently employs autologous T cells of patients for CAR expression. The autologous T cells once modified with CAR vectors ex vivo are infused back into the patient. The major advantage of using autologous T cells versus donor-derived allogeneic T cells for CAR therapy is avoidance of MHC alloreaction and transplant rejection mediated by recipient T cells, NK cells, or antibodies. The use of cancer patient-derived T cells for CAR therapy comes with several challenges including their weaker proliferation and activation capacity in ex vivo cultures. In some cases, patient peripheral blood may yield greatly diminished number of T cells. In addition, rapid disease progression and shorter timeline for treatment requirements can impose significant challenges in manufacturing "on demand" autologous CAR-T products. Utilizing healthy donor-derived allogeneic T cells could provide greater flexibility and greater efficiency in manufacturing clinical grade CAR-T products after thorough in vitro and in vivo testing. Moreover, allogenic CARs could provide greater flexibility in manufacturing clinical grade CAR-T products against various cancers that could be made available "on demand" for cancer treatment. If transplant rejection due to MHC mismatch can be controlled, allogenic CAR can be universally applied. Some early studies in the direction of manufacturing "Universal CARs" have been reported. Donor-derived CAR-T cells possess endogenous $\alpha\beta$-T cell receptor ($\alpha\beta$-TCR) that could react with recipient MHC haplotypes to trigger graft versus host disease and can quickly cause rejection of infused CAR-T cells. Therefore, deletion of endogenous αβ-TCR on donor CAR-T-modified and unmodified T cells in the graft can eliminate graft versus host response. Torikai et al. in their study, confirmed the feasibility of this approach. Utilizing zinc finger nucleases (ZFNs) to mediate precise genome editing through catalyzing double-strand DNA breaks on αβ-TCR locus in donor-derived T cells. These were subsequently genetically modified to express anti-CD19 CAR [138]. They further demonstrated that αβ-TCR^{neg} CD19 CARs maintained tumor cytotoxicity and abolished graft versus host disease. Similarly, Qasim et al. reported manufacturing and application of allogenic anti-CD19 CAR with deleted α-TCR chain and *CD52* gene loci for the treatment of two infants with refractory B-ALL. They utilized transcription activator-like effector nuclease (TALEN) gene editing enzyme to delete B-ALL patient endogenous α-TCR and *CD52* gene loci. They first applied TALEN to delete *CD52* gene to enhance the survival of T cells in the presence of Alemtuzumab. Alemtuzumab is a humanized antibody that binds to CD52 antigen to mediate lymphodepletion. Following the *CD52* gene deletion, they performed lentiviral infection on CD52^{neg} T cells to express anti-CD19 CAR, following which they electroporated a second set of TALEN enzyme to delete α-TCR chain gene locus [139]. By this approach, they reported 99% depletion of endogenous TCRs in CAR-modified T cells and were able to generate resistance to alemtuzumab as well as achieved long-term remission and in vivo CAR persistence. It is important to note that despite complete deletion of αβ-TCR, donor non-T-cell contamination can leave host cells vulnerable to NK-mediated lysis. In addition, NK cell missing-self-response against lack of MHC class I may cause destruction of allogenic CAR-T cells. MHC I molecule is not expressed on resting T cells. Gornalusse et al. demonstrated that *HLA-E* knockin at Beta-2 Microglobulin (B2M) gene locus disrupted all MHC-class I expression and provided resistance against NK-cell-mediated killing [140]. Therefore, utilizing genome-editing technology to knockin *HLA-E* gene at Beta-2 Microglobulin (B2M) gene locus can completely abolish NK cell missing self-response against allogeneic CAR-T cells.

As clear from the discussion above significant challenges remain in the realization of universal CARs, but with the new technological advances these challenges will be eventually overcome. Apart from scientific challenges, overcoming commercial and industrial interests as well as cost of manufacturing CAR products remains much bigger challenges in harnessing full potential of CAR therapy. CAR therapy is driven in part by the industrial and commercial interests. Therefore, purely from the business angle, CAR therapy will be directed toward the cancers that have significant prevalence, and refractory to available treatments. Therefore, manufacturing CARs to treat rare cancers may not be commercially a viable option that unfortunately means that some of the rare cancers will not be tested for CAR treatment in foreseeable future. The concept of designing Universal CARs have potential to greatly lower the cost associated with CAR manufacturing that eventually could benefit greater number of patients with cancers.

REFERENCES

[1] Fitzgerald JC, Weiss SL, Maude SL, Barrett DM, Lacey SF, Melenhorst JJ, et al. Cytokine release syndrome after chimeric antigen receptor T cell therapy for acute lymphoblastic leukemia. Crit Care Med 2017;45:e124−31.
[2] Abe BT, Shin DS, Mocholi E, Macian F. NFAT1 supports tumor-induced anergy of CD4(+) T cells. Cancer Res 2012;72:4642−51.
[3] Martinez GJ, Pereira RM, Aijo T, Kim EY, Marangoni F, Pipkin ME, et al. The transcription factor NFAT promotes exhaustion of activated CD8(+) T cells. Immunity 2015;42:265−78.
[4] Mognol GP, Spreafico R, Wong V, Scott-Browne JP, Togher S, Hoffmann A, et al. Exhaustion-associated regulatory regions in CD8(+) tumor-infiltrating T cells. Proc Natl Acad Sci USA 2017;114:E2776−85.
[5] Zajac AJ, Blattman JN, Murali-Krishna K, Sourdive DJ, Suresh M, Altman JD, et al. Viral immune evasion due to persistence of activated T cells without effector function. J Exp Med 1998;188:2205−13.
[6] Wherry EJ. T cell exhaustion. Nat Immunol 2011;12:492−9.
[7] Balkhi MY, Wittmann G, Xiong F, Junghans RP. YY1 upregulates checkpoint receptors and downregulates type I cytokines in exhausted, chronically stimulated human T cells. iScience 2018;2:105−22.
[8] Alfei F, Zehn D. T cell exhaustion: an epigenetically imprinted phenotypic and functional makeover. Trends Mol Med 2017;23:769−71.
[9] Man K, Gabriel SS, Liao Y, Gloury R, Preston S, Henstridge DC, et al. Transcription factor IRF4 promotes CD8(+) T cell exhaustion and limits the development of memory-like T cells during chronic infection. Immunity 2017;47:1129−11241 e5.
[10] Chihara N, Madi A, Kondo T, Zhang H, Acharya N, Singer M, et al. Induction and transcriptional regulation of the co-inhibitory gene module in T cells. Nature 2018;558:454−9.
[11] Maude SL, Teachey DT, Rheingold SR, Shaw PA, Aplenc R, Barrett DM, et al. Sustained remissions with CD19-specific chimeric antigen receptor (CAR)-modified T cells in children with relapsed/refractory ALL. J Clin Oncol 2016;34:3011.

[12] Park JH, Riviere I, Gonen M, Wang X, Senechal B, Curran KJ, et al. Long-term follow-up of CD19 CAR therapy in acute lymphoblastic leukemia. N Engl J Med 2018;378:449−59.

[13] Long AH, Haso WM, Shern JF, Wanhainen KM, Murgai M, Ingaramo M, et al. 4-1BB costimulation ameliorates T cell exhaustion induced by tonic signaling of chimeric antigen receptors. Nat Med 2015;21:581−90.

[14] Cherkassky L, Morello A, Villena-Vargas J, Feng Y, Dimitrov DS, Jones DR, et al. Human CAR T cells with cell-intrinsic PD-1 checkpoint blockade resist tumor-mediated inhibition. J Clin Invest 2016;126:3130−44.

[15] John LB, Devaud C, Duong CP, Yong CS, Beavis PA, Haynes NM, et al. Anti-PD-1 antibody therapy potently enhances the eradication of established tumors by gene-modified T cells. Clin Cancer Res 2013;19:5636−46.

[16] Zolov SN, Rietberg SP, Bonifant CL. Programmed cell death protein 1 activation preferentially inhibits CD28.CAR-T cells. Cytotherapy 2018;20:1259−66.

[17] Baitsch L, Baumgaertner P, Devevre E, Raghav SK, Legat A, Barba L, et al. Exhaustion of tumor-specific CD8(+) T cells in metastases from melanoma patients. J Clin Investig 2011;121:2350−60.

[18] Balkhi MY, Ma Q, Ahmad S, Junghans RP. T cell exhaustion and Interleukin 2 downregulation. Cytokine 2015; 71:339−47.

[19] Rosenberg SA, Mule JJ, Spiess PJ, Reichert CM, Schwarz SL. Regression of established pulmonary metastases and subcutaneous tumor mediated by the systemic administration of high-dose recombinant interleukin 2. J Exp Med 1985;161:1169−88.

[20] Blattman JN, Grayson JM, Wherry EJ, Kaech SM, Smith KA, Ahmed R. Therapeutic use of IL-2 to enhance antiviral T-cell responses in vivo. Nat Med 2003;9:540−7.

[21] Emtage PC, Lo AS, Gomes EM, Liu DL, Gonzalo-Daganzo RM, Junghans RP. Second-generation anti-carcinoembryonic antigen designer T cells resist activation-induced cell death, proliferate on tumor contact, secrete cytokines, and exhibit superior antitumor activity in vivo: a preclinical evaluation. Clin Cancer Res 2008;14:8112−22.

[22] Lo AS, Ma Q, Liu DL, Junghans RP. Anti-GD3 chimeric sFv-CD28/T-cell receptor zeta designer T cells for treatment of metastatic melanoma and other neuroectodermal tumors. Clin Cancer Res 2010;16:2769−80.

[23] Liao W, Lin JX, Leonard WJ. Interleukin-2 at the crossroads of effector responses, tolerance, and immunotherapy. Immunity 2013;38:13−25.

[24] Kershaw MH, Westwood JA, Parker LL, Wang G, Eshhar Z, Mavroukakis SA, et al. A phase I study on adoptive immunotherapy using gene-modified T cells for ovarian cancer. Clin Cancer Res 2006;12:6106−15.

[25] Lamers CH, Sleijfer S, van Steenbergen S, van Elzakker P, van Krimpen B, Groot C, et al. Treatment of metastatic renal cell carcinoma with CAIX CAR-engineered T cells: clinical evaluation and management of on-target toxicity. Mol Ther 2013;21:904−12.

[26] Fraietta JA, Lacey SF, Orlando EJ, Pruteanu-Malinici I, Gohil M, Lundh S, et al. Determinants of response and resistance to CD19 chimeric antigen receptor (CAR) T cell therapy of chronic lymphocytic leukemia. Nat Med 2018;24:563−71.

[27] Fry TJ, Mackall CL. Interleukin-7: master regulator of peripheral T-cell homeostasis? Trends Immunol 2001;22: 564−71.

[28] Bradley LM, Haynes L, Swain SL. IL-7: maintaining T-cell memory and achieving homeostasis. Trends Immunol 2005;26:172−6.

[29] Adachi K, Kano Y, Nagai T, Okuyama N, Sakoda Y, Tamada K. IL-7 and CCL19 expression in CAR-T cells improves immune cell infiltration and CAR-T cell survival in the tumor. Nat Biotechnol 2018;36:346−51.

[30] Burga RA, Thorn M, Point GR, Guha P, Nguyen CT, Licata LA, et al. Liver myeloid-derived suppressor cells expand in response to liver metastases in mice and inhibit the anti-tumor efficacy of anti-CEA CAR-T. Cancer Immunol Immunother 2015;64:817−29.

[31] Gargett T, Yu W, Dotti G, Yvon ES, Christo SN, Hayball JD, et al. GD2-specific CAR T cells undergo potent activation and deletion following antigen encounter but can be protected from activation-induced cell death by PD-1 blockade. Mol Ther 2016; 24:1135−49.

[32] Liu X, Ranganathan R, Jiang S, Fang C, Sun J, Kim S, et al. A chimeric switch-receptor targeting PD1 augments the efficacy of second-generation CAR T cells in advanced solid tumors. Cancer Res 2016;76:1578−90.

[33] June CH, O'Connor RS, Kawalekar OU, Ghassemi S, Milone MC. CAR T cell immunotherapy for human cancer. Science 2018;359:1361−5.

[34] Lugli E, Dominguez MH, Gattinoni L, Chattopadhyay PK, Bolton DL, Song K, et al. Superior T memory stem cell persistence supports long-lived T cell memory. J Clin Investig 2013;123:594−9.

[35] Zhang X, Sun S, Hwang I, Tough DF, Sprent J. Potent and selective stimulation of memory-phenotype CD8+ T cells in vivo by IL-15. Immunity 1998;8:591−9.

[36] Lodolce J, Burkett P, Koka R, Boone D, Chien M, Chan F, et al. Interleukin-15 and the regulation of lymphoid homeostasis. Mol Immunol 2002;39:537−44.

[37] Lodolce JP, Burkett PR, Koka RM, Boone DL, Ma A. Regulation of lymphoid homeostasis by interleukin-15. Cytokine Growth Factor Rev 2002;13:429−39.

[38] Cheever MA. Twelve immunotherapy drugs that could cure cancers. Immunol Rev 2008;222:357−68.

[39] Dadi S, Chhangawala S, Whitlock BM, Franklin RA, Luo CT, Oh SA, et al. Cancer immunosurveillance by tissue-resident innate lymphoid cells and innate-like T cells. Cell 2016;164:365−77.

[40] Citro G, Perrotti D, Cucco C, D'Agnano I, Sacchi A, Zupi G, et al. Inhibition of leukemia cell proliferation by receptor-mediated uptake of c-myb antisense oligodeoxynucleotides. Proc Natl Acad Sci USA 1992; 89:7031−5.

[41] Rubinstein MP, Kovar M, Purton JF, Cho JH, Boyman O, Surh CD, et al. Converting IL-15 to a superagonist by binding to soluble IL-15R{alpha}. Proc Natl Acad Sci USA 2006;103:9166−71.

[42] Hurton LV, Singh H, Najjar AM, Switzer KC, Mi T, Maiti S, et al. Tethered IL-15 augments antitumor activity and promotes a stem-cell memory subset in tumor-specific T cells. Proc Natl Acad Sci USA 2016;113: E7788−97.

[43] Di Stasi A, De Angelis B, Rooney CM, Zhang L, Mahendravada A, Foster AE, et al. T lymphocytes coexpressing CCR4 and a chimeric antigen receptor targeting CD30 have improved homing and antitumor activity in a Hodgkin tumor model. Blood 2009;113:6392−402.

[44] Tschumi BO, Dumauthioz N, Marti B, Zhang L, Schneider P, Mach JP, et al. CART cells are prone to Fas- and DR5-mediated cell death. J Immunother Cancer 2018;6:71.

[45] Boise LH, Gonzalez-Garcia M, Postema CE, Ding L, Lindsten T, Turka LA, et al. bcl-x, a bcl-2-related gene that functions as a dominant regulator of apoptotic cell death. Cell 1993;74:597−608.

[46] Michels J, Kepp O, Senovilla L, Lissa D, Castedo M, Kroemer G, et al. Functions of BCL-X L at the interface between cell death and metabolism. Int J Cell Biol 2013;2013:705294.

[47] Schulze-Bergkamen H, Krammer PH. Apoptosis in cancer–implications for therapy. Semin Oncol 2004;31: 90−119.

[48] Boise LH, Noel PJ, Thompson CB. CD28 and apoptosis. Curr Opin Immunol 1995;7:620−5.

[49] Boise LH, Minn AJ, Noel PJ, June CH, Accavitti MA, Lindsten T, et al. CD28 costimulation can promote T cell survival by enhancing the expression of Bcl-XL. Immunity 1995;3:87−98.

[50] Wu LX, La Rose J, Chen L, Neale C, Mak T, Okkenhaug K, et al. CD28 regulates the translation of Bcl-xL via the phosphatidylinositol 3-kinase/mammalian target of rapamycin pathway. J Immunol 2005;174:180−94.

[51] Krammer PH. CD95(APO-1/Fas)-mediated apoptosis: live and let die. Adv Immunol 1999;71:163−210.

[52] Waring P, Mullbacher A. Cell death induced by the Fas/Fas ligand pathway and its role in pathology. Immunol Cell Biol 1999;77:312−7.

[53] Charo J, Robbins PF. Contrasting effects of FLIPL overexpression in human T cells on activation-induced cell death and cytokine production. J Leukoc Biol 2007;81: 1297−302.

[54] Brentjens RJ, Davila ML, Riviere I, Park J, Wang X, Cowell LG, et al. CD19-targeted T cells rapidly induce molecular remissions in adults with chemotherapy-refractory acute lymphoblastic leukemia. Sci Transl Med 2013;5:177ra38.

[55] Grupp SA, Kalos M, Barrett D, Aplenc R, Porter DL, Rheingold SR, et al. Chimeric antigen receptor-modified T cells for acute lymphoid leukemia. N Engl J Med 2013;368:1509−18.

[56] Porter DL, Levine BL, Kalos M, Bagg A, June CH. Chimeric antigen receptor-modified T cells in chronic lymphoid leukemia. N Engl J Med 2011;365:725−33.

[57] Otero DC, Rickert RC. CD19 function in early and late B cell development. II. CD19 facilitates the pro-B/pre-B transition. J Immunol 2003;171:5921−30.

[58] Cariappa A, Boboila C, Moran ST, Liu H, Shi HN, Pillai S. The recirculating B cell pool contains two functionally distinct, long-lived, posttransitional, follicular B cell populations. J Immunol 2007;179:2270−81.

[59] Cariappa A, Chase C, Liu H, Russell P, Pillai S. Naive recirculating B cells mature simultaneously in the spleen and bone marrow. Blood 2007;109:2339−45.

[60] Cariappa A, Tang M, Parng C, Nebelitskiy E, Carroll M, Georgopoulos K, et al. The follicular versus marginal zone B lymphocyte cell fate decision is regulated by Aiolos, Btk, and CD21. Immunity 2001;14:603−15.

[61] Dunn GP, Old LJ, Schreiber RD. The three Es of cancer immunoediting. Annu Rev Immunol 2004;22:329−60.

[62] Maude SL, Laetsch TW, Buechner J, Rives S, Boyer M, Bittencourt H, et al. Tisagenlecleucel in children and young adults with B-cell lymphoblastic leukemia. N Engl J Med 2018;378:439−48.

[63] Zhang T, Cao L, Xie J, Shi N, Zhang Z, Luo Z, et al. Efficiency of CD19 chimeric antigen receptor-modified T cells for treatment of B cell malignancies in phase I clinical trials: a meta-analysis. Oncotarget 2015;6: 33961−71.

[64] Evans AG, Rothberg PG, Burack WR, Huntington SF, Porter DL, Friedberg JW, et al. Evolution to plasmablastic lymphoma evades CD19-directed chimeric antigen receptor T cells. Br J Haematol 2015;171:205−9.

[65] Sotillo E, Barrett DM, Black KL, Bagashev A, Oldridge D, Wu G, et al. Convergence of acquired mutations and alternative splicing of CD19 enables resistance to CART-19 immunotherapy. Cancer Discov 2015;5: 1282−95.

[66] Hegde M, Corder A, Chow KK, Mukherjee M, Ashoori A, Kew Y, et al. Combinational targeting offsets antigen escape and enhances effector functions of adoptively transferred T cells in glioblastoma. Mol Ther 2013;21: 2087−101.

[67] Kent SJ, Greenberg PD, Hoffman MC, Akridge RE, McElrath MJ. Antagonism of vaccine-induced HIV-1-specific CD4$^+$ T cells by primary HIV-1 infection: potential mechanism of vaccine failure. J Immunol 1997;158: 807−15.

[68] Zhang YM, Imamichi H, Imamichi T, Lane HC, Falloon J, Vasudevachari MB, et al. Drug resistance during indinavir therapy is caused by mutations in the protease gene and in its Gag substrate cleavage sites. J Virol 1997;71:6662−70.

[69] Fry TJ, Shah NN, Orentas RJ, Stetler-Stevenson M, Yuan CM, Ramakrishna S, et al. CD22-targeted CAR T cells induce remission in B-ALL that is naive or resistant to CD19-targeted CAR immunotherapy. Nat Med 2018;24:20−8.

[70] Ali SA, Shi V, Maric I, Wang M, Stroncek DF, Rose JJ, et al. T cells expressing an anti-B-cell maturation antigen chimeric antigen receptor cause remissions of multiple myeloma. Blood 2016;128:1688—700.

[71] Long AH, Haso WM, Orentas RJ. Lessons learned from a highly-active CD22-specific chimeric antigen receptor. Oncoimmunology 2013;2:e23621.

[72] Doody GM, Justement LB, Delibrias CC, Matthews RJ, Lin J, Thomas ML, et al. A role in B cell activation for CD22 and the protein tyrosine phosphatase SHP. Science 1995;269:242—4.

[73] Jellusova J, Nitschke L. Regulation of B cell functions by the sialic acid-binding receptors siglec-G and CD22. Front Immunol 2011;2:96.

[74] Martyniszyn A, Krahl AC, Andre MC, Hombach AA, Abken H. CD20-CD19 bispecific CAR T cells for the treatment of B-cell malignancies. Hum Gene Ther 2017;28:1147—57.

[75] Nolan KF, Yun CO, Akamatsu Y, Murphy JC, Leung SO, Beecham EJ, et al. Bypassing immunization: optimized design of "designer T cells" against carcinoembryonic antigen (CEA)-expressing tumors, and lack of suppression by soluble CEA. Clin Cancer Res 1999;5:3928—41.

[76] Arndt C, Feldmann A, Koristka S, Cartellieri M, Dimmel M, Ehninger A, et al. Simultaneous targeting of prostate stem cell antigen and prostate-specific membrane antigen improves the killing of prostate cancer cells using a novel modular T cell-retargeting system. Prostate 2014;74:1335—46.

[77] Yaghoubi SS, Jensen MC, Satyamurthy N, Budhiraja S, Paik D, Czernin J, et al. Noninvasive detection of therapeutic cytolytic T cells with 18F—FHBG PET in a patient with glioma. Nat Clin Pract Oncol 2008;6:53.

[78] Keu KV, Witney TH, Yaghoubi S, Rosenberg J, Kurien A, Magnusson R, et al. Reporter gene imaging of targeted T cell immunotherapy in recurrent glioma. Sci Transl Med 2017;9.

[79] Matz MV, Fradkov AF, Labas YA, Savitsky AP, Zaraisky AG, Markelov ML, et al. Fluorescent proteins from nonbioluminescent Anthozoa species. Nat Biotechnol 1999;17:969—73.

[80] Sommermeyer D, Hill T, Shamah SM, Salter AI, Chen Y, Mohler KM, et al. Fully human CD19-specific chimeric antigen receptors for T-cell therapy. Leukemia 2017;31: 2191—9.

[81] Kalos M, Levine BL, Porter DL, Katz S, Grupp SA, Bagg A, et al. T cells with chimeric antigen receptors have potent antitumor effects and can establish memory in patients with advanced leukemia. Sci Transl Med 2011;3:95ra73.

[82] Cheung A, Bax HJ, Josephs DH, Ilieva KM, Pellizzari G, Opzoomer J, et al. Targeting folate receptor alpha for cancer treatment. Oncotarget 2016;7:52553—74.

[83] authors N. Regulating CAR T cells: a remote control approach. Cancer Discov 2016;6:936—7.

[84] Teachey DT, Lacey SF, Shaw PA, Melenhorst JJ, Maude SL, Frey N, et al. Identification of predictive biomarkers for cytokine release syndrome after chimeric antigen receptor T-cell therapy for acute lymphoblastic leukemia. Cancer Discov 2016;6:664—79.

[85] Maude SL, Frey N, Shaw PA, Aplenc R, Barrett DM, Bunin NJ, et al. Chimeric antigen receptor T cells for sustained remissions in leukemia. N Engl J Med 2014;371: 1507—17.

[86] Teachey DT, Rheingold SR, Maude SL, Zugmaier G, Barrett DM, Seif AE, et al. Cytokine release syndrome after blinatumomab treatment related to abnormal macrophage activation and ameliorated with cytokine-directed therapy. Blood 2013;121:5154—7.

[87] Klinger M, Brandl C, Zugmaier G, Hijazi Y, Bargou RC, Topp MS, et al. Immunopharmacologic response of patients with B-lineage acute lymphoblastic leukemia to continuous infusion of T cell-engaging CD19/CD3-bispecific BiTE antibody blinatumomab. Blood 2012; 119:6226—33.

[88] Kochenderfer JN, Dudley ME, Feldman SA, Wilson WH, Spaner DE, Maric I, et al. B-cell depletion and remissions of malignancy along with cytokine-associated toxicity in a clinical trial of anti-CD19 chimeric-antigen-receptor-transduced T cells. Blood 2012;119:2709—20.

[89] Schiller JH, Storer BE, Witt PL, Alberti D, Tombes MB, Arzoomanian R, et al. Biological and clinical effects of intravenous tumor necrosis factor administered three times weekly. Cancer Res 1991;51:1651—8.

[90] Fiedler W, Zeller W, Peimann CJ, Weh HJ, Hossfeld DK. A phase II combination trial with recombinant human tumor necrosis factor and gamma interferon in patients with colorectal cancer. Klin Wochenschr 1991;69:261—8.

[91] Foon KA, Sherwin SA, Abrams PG, Stevenson HC, Holmes P, Maluish AE, et al. A phase I trial of recombinant gamma interferon in patients with cancer. Cancer Immunol Immunother 1985;20:193—7.

[92] Campana D, Schwarz H, Imai C. 4-1BB chimeric antigen receptors. Cancer J 2014;20:134—40.

[93] Tang Y, Xu X, Song H, Yang S, Shi S, Wei J, et al. Early diagnostic and prognostic significance of a specific Th1/Th2 cytokine pattern in children with haemophagocytic syndrome. Br J Haematol 2008;143:84—91.

[94] Risma K, Jordan MB. Hemophagocytic lymphohistiocytosis: updates and evolving concepts. Curr Opin Pediatr 2012;24:9—15.

[95] Barrett DM, Teachey DT, Grupp SA. Toxicity management for patients receiving novel T-cell engaging therapies. Curr Opin Pediatr 2014;26:43—9.

[96] Janka GE. Familial hemophagocytic lymphohistiocytosis. Eur J Pediatr 1983;140:221—30.

[97] Gust J, Hay KA, Hanafi LA, Li D, Myerson D, Gonzalez-Cuyar LF, et al. Endothelial activation and blood-brain barrier disruption in neurotoxicity after adoptive immunotherapy with CD19 CAR-T cells. Cancer Discov 2017; 7:1404—19.

[98] Neelapu SS, Tummala S, Kebriaei P, Wierda W, Gutierrez C, Locke FL, et al. Chimeric antigen receptor T-cell therapy - assessment and management of toxicities. Nat Rev Clin Oncol 2018;15:47—62.

[99] Geyer MB, Riviere I, Senechal B, Wang X, Wang Y, Purdon TJ, et al. Autologous CD19-targeted CAR T cells in patients with residual CLL following initial purine analog-based therapy. Mol Ther 2018;26: 1896—905.

[100] Turtle CJ, Hanafi LA, Berger C, Hudecek M, Pender B, Robinson E, et al. Immunotherapy of non-Hodgkin's lymphoma with a defined ratio of CD8+ and CD4+ CD19-specific chimeric antigen receptor-modified T cells. Sci Transl Med 2016;8:355ra116.

[101] Davila ML, Riviere I, Wang X, Bartido S, Park J, Curran K, et al. Efficacy and toxicity management of 19-28z CAR T cell therapy in B cell acute lymphoblastic leukemia. Sci Transl Med 2014;6:224ra25.

[102] Taraseviciute A, Tkachev V, Ponce R, Turtle CJ, Snyder JM, Liggitt HD, et al. Chimeric antigen receptor T cell-mediated neurotoxicity in nonhuman primates. Cancer Discov 2018;8:750—63.

[103] Heinrich PC, Behrmann I, Muller-Newen G, Schaper F, Graeve L. Interleukin-6-type cytokine signalling through the gp130/Jak/STAT pathway. Biochem J 1998;334(Pt 2):297—314.

[104] Schett G. Physiological effects of modulating the interleukin-6 axis. Rheumatology (Oxford) 2018;57: ii43—50.

[105] Gallipoli P. JAK of all trades: ruxolitinib as a new therapeutic option for CML patients. Leuk Res 2018;75:71—2.

[106] Singh JA, Wells GA, Christensen R, Tanjong Ghogomu E, Maxwell L, Macdonald JK, et al. Adverse effects of biologics: a network meta-analysis and Cochrane overview. Cochrane Database Syst Rev 2011:CD008794.

[107] Woo P, Wilkinson N, Prieur AM, Southwood T, Leone V, Livermore P, et al. Open label phase II trial of single, ascending doses of MRA in Caucasian children with severe systemic juvenile idiopathic arthritis: proof of principle of the efficacy of IL-6 receptor blockade in this type of arthritis and demonstration of prolonged clinical improvement. Arthritis Res Ther 2005;7:R1281—8.

[108] Yokota S, Miyamae T, Imagawa T, Iwata N, Katakura S, Mori M, et al. Therapeutic efficacy of humanized recombinant anti-interleukin-6 receptor antibody in children with systemic-onset juvenile idiopathic arthritis. Arthritis Rheum 2005;52:818—25.

[109] De Benedetti F, Brunner HI, Ruperto N, Kenwright A, Wright S, Calvo I, et al. Randomized trial of tocilizumab in systemic juvenile idiopathic arthritis. N Engl J Med 2012;367:2385—95.

[110] Norelli M, Camisa B, Barbiera G, Falcone L, Purevdorj A, Genua M, et al. Monocyte-derived IL-1 and IL-6 are differentially required for cytokine-release syndrome and neurotoxicity due to CAR T cells. Nat Med 2018; 24:739—48.

[111] Tomaske M, Amon O, Bosk A, Handgretinger R, Schneider EM, Niethammer D. Alpha-CD25 antibody treatment in a child with hemophagocytic lymphohistiocytosis. Med Pediatr Oncol 2002;38: 141—2.

[112] Giavridis T, van der Stegen SJC, Eyquem J, Hamieh M, Piersigilli A, Sadelain M. CAR T cell-induced cytokine release syndrome is mediated by macrophages and abated by IL-1 blockade. Nat Med 2018;24:731—8.

[113] Lee DW, Kochenderfer JN, Stetler-Stevenson M, Cui YK, Delbrook C, Feldman SA, et al. T cells expressing CD19 chimeric antigen receptors for acute lymphoblastic leukaemia in children and young adults: a phase 1 dose-escalation trial. Lancet 2015;385:517—28.

[114] Mahadeo KM, Khazal SJ, Abdel-Azim H, Fitzgerald JC, Taraseviciute A, Bollard CM, et al. Management guidelines for paediatric patients receiving chimeric antigen receptor T cell therapy. Nat Rev Clin Oncol 2018;16: 45—63.

[115] Liu X, Zhang N, Shi H. Driving better and safer HER2-specific CARs for cancer therapy. Oncotarget 2017;8: 62730—41.

[116] Morgan RA, Yang JC, Kitano M, Dudley ME, Laurencot CM, Rosenberg SA. Case report of a serious adverse event following the administration of T cells transduced with a chimeric antigen receptor recognizing ERBB2. Mol Ther 2010;18:843—51.

[117] Kameda T, Yasui W, Yoshida K, Tsujino T, Nakayama H, Ito M, et al. Expression of ERBB2 in human gastric carcinomas: relationship between p185ERBB2 expression and the gene amplification. Cancer Res 1990;50:8002—9.

[118] Slamon DJ, Godolphin W, Jones LA, Holt JA, Wong SG, Keith DE, et al. Studies of the HER-2/neu protooncogene in human breast and ovarian cancer. Science 1989;244:707—12.

[119] Yarden Y, Shilo BZ. SnapShot: EGFR signaling pathway. Cell 2007;131:1018.

[120] Richman SA, Nunez-Cruz S, Moghimi B, Li LZ, Gershenson ZT, Mourelatos Z, et al. High-affinity GD2-specific CAR T cells induce fatal encephalitis in a preclinical neuroblastoma model. Cancer Immunol Res 2018;6:36—46.

[121] Hoyos V, Savoldo B, Quintarelli C, Mahendravada A, Zhang M, Vera J, et al. Engineering CD19-specific T lymphocytes with interleukin-15 and a suicide gene to enhance their anti-lymphoma/leukemia effects and safety. Leukemia 2010;24:1160—70.

[122] Gargett T, Brown MP. The inducible caspase-9 suicide gene system as a "safety switch" to limit on-target, off-tumor toxicities of chimeric antigen receptor T cells. Front Pharmacol 2014;5:235.

[123] Robbins PF, Lu YC, El-Gamil M, Li YF, Gross C, Gartner J, et al. Mining exomic sequencing data to identify mutated antigens recognized by adoptively transferred tumor-reactive T cells. Nat Med 2013;19:747—52.

[124] Lu YC, Yao X, Crystal JS, Li YF, El-Gamil M, Gross C, et al. Efficient identification of mutated cancer antigens recognized by T cells associated with durable tumor regressions. Clin Cancer Res 2014;20:3401—10.

[125] Coulie PG, Van den Eynde BJ, van der Bruggen P, Boon T. Tumour antigens recognized by T lymphocytes: at the core of cancer immunotherapy. Nat Rev Cancer 2014;14:135—46.

[126] Stevanovic S, Pasetto A, Helman SR, Gartner JJ, Prickett TD, Howie B, et al. Landscape of immunogenic tumor antigens in successful immunotherapy of virally induced epithelial cancer. Science 2017;356:200−5.

[127] Perrotti D, Jamieson C, Goldman J, Skorski T. Chronic myeloid leukemia: mechanisms of blastic transformation. J Clin Investig 2010;120:2254−64.

[128] Bjorklund AK, Forkel M, Picelli S, Konya V, Theorell J, Friberg D, et al. The heterogeneity of human CD127(+) innate lymphoid cells revealed by single-cell RNA sequencing. Nat Immunol 2016;17:451−60.

[129] Villani AC, Shekhar K. Single-cell RNA sequencing of human T cells. Methods Mol Biol 2017;1514:203−39.

[130] Proserpio V, Piccolo A, Haim-Vilmovsky L, Kar G, Lonnberg T, Svensson V, et al. Single-cell analysis of CD4$^+$ T-cell differentiation reveals three major cell states and progressive acceleration of proliferation. Genome Biol 2016;17:103.

[131] Chen YT, Gure AO, Tsang S, Stockert E, Jager E, Knuth A, et al. Identification of multiple cancer/testis antigens by allogeneic antibody screening of a melanoma cell line library. Proc Natl Acad Sci USA 1998;95:6919−23.

[132] Patel K, Olivares S, Singh H, Hurton LV, Huls MH, Qazilbash MH, et al. Combination immunotherapy with NY-ESO-1-Specific CAR$^+$ T cells with T-cell vaccine improves anti-myeloma effect. Blood 2016;128:3366.

[133] Singh N, Kulikovskaya I, Barrett DM, Binder-Scholl G, Jakobsen B, Martinez D, et al. T cells targeting NY-ESO-1 demonstrate efficacy against disseminated neuroblastoma. Oncoimmunology 2016;5:e1040216.

[134] Kuijk LM, Verstege MI, Rekers NV, Bruijns SC, Hooijberg E, Roep BO, et al. Notch controls generation and function of human effector CD8$^+$ T cells. Blood 2013;121:2638−46.

[135] Yuan JS, Kousis PC, Suliman S, Visan I, Guidos CJ. Functions of notch signaling in the immune system: consensus and controversies. Annu Rev Immunol 2010;28:343−65.

[136] Morsut L, Roybal KT, Xiong X, Gordley RM, Coyle SM, Thomson M, et al. Engineering customized cell sensing and response behaviors using synthetic notch receptors. Cell 2016;164:780−91.

[137] Roybal KT, Rupp LJ, Morsut L, Walker WJ, McNally KA, Park JS, et al. Precision tumor recognition by T cells with combinatorial antigen-sensing circuits. Cell 2016;164:770−9.

[138] Torikai H, Reik A, Liu PQ, Zhou Y, Zhang L, Maiti S, et al. A foundation for universal T-cell based immunotherapy: T cells engineered to express a CD19-specific chimeric-antigen-receptor and eliminate expression of endogenous TCR. Blood 2012;119:5697−705.

[139] Qasim W, Zhan H, Samarasinghe S, Adams S, Amrolia P, Stafford S, et al. Molecular remission of infant B-ALL after infusion of universal TALEN gene-edited CAR T cells. Sci Transl Med 2017;9.

[140] Gornalusse GG, Hirata RK, Funk SE, Riolobos L, Lopes VS, Manske G, et al. HLA-E-expressing pluripotent stem cells escape allogeneic responses and lysis by NK cells. Nat Biotechnol 2017;35:765.

Index

Note: Page numbers followed by "t" indicate tables and "f" indicate figures.

Printed in the United States
By Bookmasters